Fading Image

Mary Ray Birdwell

Published by Live Love Learn Books Publishing
LiveLoveLearnBooks.com
Cover design / book formatting by Cindy Shtevi
CindyShtevi.com
Fading Image
Copyright © 2016 by Mary Ray Birdwell
All rights reserved

Photography by Mindy Stevens
Printed in the United States of America

Library of Congress Control Number: 2016932406

ISBN-10:0-9903044-6-9
ISBN-13:978-0-9903044-6-3

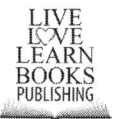

CONTENTS

Dedication

I want to dedicate "Fading Image" to anyone who ever showed my mother patience, love and kindness while she was ill with Alzheimer's. Her disease taught me more about love than anything I have experienced in my life. I received incredible support every day that she and I fought the monster, Alzheimer's. I want to thank my Facebook friends who answered all of my concerns when I would write about them. You will never know how many nights I re-read the kind messages you posted in reply to my hurts. I want to thank Patsy and Barbara for all of the Christmas cards they sent Mom, and the pajamas they sent her every Christmas. I want to thank all of the caregivers sent to watch over Mom when Mindy and I could not. I want to thank a female police officer that reminds me so much of the younger version of Mom, Diana Bell of the Rowlett Police Department. You were so kind to follow up with us. I want to thank another police officer from Argyle, Texas, who 'just happened' to listen to a little voice inside his head that fateful morning on February 11, 2010. He found mom on the railroad tracks and saved her life. I want to thank the court investigator, Adult Protection Services, and the court system, for making the right decision about Mom's guardianship. I want to thank all those who came to Mom's 78th birthday party. This is the day she seemed to be her well self and I believe it was due to all the love in the room. I want to thank Obie Ezechi for calling Mom his "Princess" and taking an extra interest in not only nursing her, but also loving her on her especially rude and bad days. I want to thank the other workers at the Memory Care Center for treating Mom like a friend not just a patient. I want to thank my neighbors, David and Sheila Jayakaren, for always watching out for Mom and for coming to court to support me. In fact, I want to thank many of her neighbors for loving and caring for her and for still asking me how things are going now that she is gone. A special thank you to Mom's mail lady. Thank you for stopping me when I was visiting one day, and telling me your concerns. I want to thank all those who also had loved ones in Memory Care, and helped Mom while she was there. We were all in the same predicament, and each mother and father at the center became our own. I want to thank John for all the times he picked up the medicine for Mom because he was closer to the pharmacy than anyone else. Thanks for staying and having breakfast with her at times. I want to thank Nico for helping me clean her room once a week, pretending to be her boyfriend, and for loving her. I want to thank my dad for coming and seeing mom at the center and for taking all my late night phone calls. I especially want to thank my dad for coming to her funeral when he felt so out of place. I want to thank my cousin, Barbara Patterson, for working with us, the courts, and anyone else she could, to figure out Mom's finances, and how to right wrongs that had been done with her accounts. I want to thank Shannon Holt at our attorney's office, who made sure I had answers when I needed them and became a personal friend to Mindy and me. I want to thank my daughter for being part of the team we became, to save my mom. We had one goal in mind to save the woman I called Momma and the woman Mindy called Nana. I want to thank my Son-in-Law, Tony, for listening to me cry so often on the phone, not losing patience with me, and for always finding time to come and visit Mom on those special occasions at the Memory Care Unit. I want to personally thank Stephen Thompson for making the box for me to place at the bottom of the pool, and for the heart he placed in the plaster over Mom's buried things. I want to thank my publisher for pushing me after Mom died in March. I really wanted to just hide and forget everything I had ever written. The memories of Mom were overwhelming and the thought of reliving that nightmare was too much at times. She helped me to march on and to write, which was a blessing to say the least. Writing got me through the ordeal and would also help me to heal. I also want to thank the DPD for the beautiful job they did at mom's memorial. The taps they played, and the presentation of the Texas flag as they thanked me for her service, made me feel honored! I also want to thank Governor Greg Abbot for his letter of condolences and the flag that was flown over the Texas state capital. Thank you to Kim Vickers, Executive Director over Texas Commission on Law Enforcement for her letter of condolences and the Memoriam and Recognition letter. I have framed each of these and they are proudly displayed on my wall. They will be cherished.

I want to thank my counselor, Harry Cates. If not for Harry I would never have embarked on the journey to save my mom, and I would have stayed in my fear mode.

There was a job that needed to be done. It was not easy by any means. It was long, it was tedious and it was one that almost drove me to the brink of severe depression. But, in the end it would become the best decision I have ever made. It was a decision to give my mom more years with us, and to prove you have to fight for what is right and fight against what is unjust and wrong. Thank you to the most caring counselor I could ever wish to be professionally guided by.

I am sure there are many more people I could thank, and I hope I have, or will get the chance to one day. How do you ever thank someone enough for loving your mother in her most desperate time of need? *Fading Image* would never have been anything but thoughts on a piece of paper, without all of the other ingredients. God gave me unlimited access to all of His resources. HE supplied all my needs. Today, I can honestly say I am thankful for the journey with my mom through the mire of her disease, Alzheimer's.

I personally dedicate this book to a very humble woman, my mom, Rosemary Dedman Birdwell Katzen, "my mentor; my hero".

"I, the Lord, have called you to demonstrate my righteousness.
I will take you by the hand and guard you." Isaiah 42:6 NLT

Foreword

There are many thieves and many cruelties in this life, but few match the struggle of watching someone we love suffer through the degrading terminal illness of Alzheimer's. I have witnessed the journey of people struggling through the maze of dementia in its many forms both up close and from a distance. While I have been spared this in my immediate family and those closest to me, I have seen a long-time friend watch his father's decline and death from dementia. He did everything he could but knew it wasn't a winnable battle even though he is a neurologist, a cruel irony. Also, my aunt spent several years in the slow fade that is Alzheimer's. In my professional life, I have tried to help many families of people suffering with this disrespectful disease find their way through the labyrinth of their loved one's slow exit.

The story of *Fading Image* is the story of Mary and her unique journey through her mother's slow acquiescence to the terminal and relentless decline of Alzheimer's. My role in this has been as a helper and a guide to Mary and her family as they moved through Rosemary's decline. My role was small compared to the courage of a daughter to keep going through it all. It is testament to her strength and will that Mary never gave up and kept finding the small joys and humor in what is mostly a confusing and unpredictable wasteland.

Because there are many things families struggle with along the long road of dementia illnesses, the potential pitfalls are numerous. It seems appropriate to point out a small list of important things to avoid when dealing with dementia.

Remaining in denial of the dementia for months or years, and thus delaying important steps to protect and care for their loved one.

Delaying taking necessary legal steps to protect their loved one's interests, and respect their end of life wishes.

Arguing with, or trying to correct their loved one's memory as they begin to change and suffer the inevitable cognitive decompensation.

Expecting perfection from long-term care and caregivers, or not expecting enough from them.

Spending too much time visiting when they are at a point they need 24-hour care, or, just as bad, spending too little time.

Forgetting to love and respect the part of their loved one that is left until the image fades completely.

While this list could go on almost indefinitely, I believe it is of utmost importance that all who are caring for a dementia sufferer make sure to take care of themselves, as well as their loved ones. Otherwise, the caregiver will become a victim of the collateral damage of the disease. Something I believe their loved one would never want.

The intimate and vulnerable details shared in this beautiful story show one person's individual and private passage of seeing 'Mom' through the unforgiving and unrelenting illness of Alzheimer's. While every struggle and path is unique, there are many shared emotions, thoughts, and moments of the many people caring for a loved one with dementia. I hope this book will shed some new light on this terrible disease and encourage all of us to have compassion for those with dementia and their caregivers. And if you find yourself in this role, I hope you will have the strength and courage to stay strong. I hope you will ask for help when it's needed and glean from the wisdom of those who have already made this painful journey.

Harry Cates LPC

Preface

"Fading Image" started out as a blog on Facebook. It was my way of coping, an out for me. Writing has always been an integral part of my life for as long as I can remember. As a young child, with pencil and paper, I would go off into my room, preferably my closet. In the sanctuary of that very small space I felt safe to put my feelings on paper. I hoped the magic of writing about hurts could make them disappear or if nothing else make them less painful.

When my mom began asking the same question over and over again, we all became very frustrated. Having someone sit in front of you and ask you the same question five times in a thirty minute period can readily grate on one's nerves. Your frustration quickly turns into fear. The first stages of Alzheimer's with the non-sufferer are confusion, fear, helplessness, denial and sometimes anger. Now, imagine how the Alzheimer's sufferer actually feels. We, the non-sufferer can reach out for answers. The sufferer has none.

Have you ever awakened from a nightmare terribly petrified? I have. I had what is called a night terror dream. I awoke thinking I could not see; I was blind. I was in terror, half awake, half asleep. I felt like screaming aloud would not be enough to express the intense anxiety I felt. I slowly awakened and realized I was not blind, I was in my own room and I was safe. After the journey with my mom and learning more and more about the disease of Alzheimer's, I realized this might be how they feel much of the time. I think I would ask the same question too, over and over again.

I want to say, Alzheimer's was the only malady Mom had to overcome. She also endured psychological, emotional, and financial abuse. Sometimes we have to realize it can be those closest to us who can cause physical or mental damage or injury. They have a name for this today, it is called Elder Abuse. In *Fading Image* I will not dwell on this part of our journey. I will, however, mention those who helped to save my mom from her abusers. There were many beginning with caregivers, a court investigator, neuro-psychiatrist, Adult Protective Services (APS), Family law/ Probate Paralegal, Rowlett policewoman, Argyle policeman, friends, family and an extremely good counselor.

In the beginning of any journey you need someone, somewhere who can show you the way. They usually have experienced where you are going and have walked your path before. They can walk beside you and guide you through your journey. Harry Cates, a licensed counselor, was my guide. He started me on the passage of saving my mom. Although I could not save her from the cunning disease of Alzheimer's, I did help her to maintain a resemblance of some normalcy. Maybe it was more for me than for her. I knew my mom and knew it would be what she desired most, to appear normal- above all else.

She lived her last few years free of neglect, abuse, and every type of coercion.

Fading Image

In The Beginning

There is such confusion. You will be baffled. You will get angry. You may ask yourself, why is my loved one doing these things? Do they want attention? Is it a lack of sleep? Have they lost their mind, or have I lost mine? First let me say, there is a difference between asking a question twice in a day, and asking the same question five times in one day. There is also a difference in telling a story you were told, and telling the same story twice in one day. It is normal to forget where you left your car keys. It is not normal to find them in the refrigerator or forget what they are used for. There will not be *little* differences in behavior, there will be *noticeable* differences. There will be paranoia. My mom had horrible paranoia. As I look back now, someone was aiding in the feeding of her paranoia. It was a way of alienating her from family and friends. I got calls at odd hours accusing me of bringing my three children over and letting them eat cookies in her bed. I have an only child. I did not have a key to her house. The locks had been changed and not by her. My mom was having significant delusions and paranoia. She left notes all around her house and even on her front door stating she had no money and not to rob her house. She accused family members of stealing her money. Remember, this is not the norm for first stage Alzheimer's. It is however, a red flag for abuse or misuse of medication. I knew virtually nothing about this disease. I had no idea she suffered from it. I was baffled and I kept wondering why my mother had taken such a disliking to me, my daughter whom she absolutely adored and two great grandchildren she worshiped. These are not normal signs of early onset Alzheimer's when the sufferer still knows the family. These are signs of a person who is in first stage and is not being properly seen by a physician. They are not taking the correct dosage of medication and are not being told the truth. People they believe they can trust easily can mislead an Alzheimer/Dementia sufferer. Unfortunately, in the beginning my mom trusted the wrong people.

I blame myself at times when she pushed me away; I got scared and stayed away. I have great guilt about this. I was ignorant as to what she was going through. She was suffering from elder abuse and from the first stages of Alzheimer's. Two maladies in one.

On February 10, 2010 my mother was driving alone in her vehicle following someone she trusted. She had no cell phone, no change. He had a cell phone and change and full capacity of his mental abilities. Months earlier I had taken her to a Neuropsychologist where she had six hours of testing done. The second visit, the three of us closest to her attended. We were ALL told not to let her drive or to let her make any financial decisions. She was incapable of doing so. But, on this day she had been instructed to follow the man she married in 2005. Of course she got lost! My mom notified my daughter a few hours later and stated she was at a Shell gas station and had lost her way. Could we send help for her? Then the phone went dead. From the time she was lost until the police were notified it was over four hours. The police were notified first by me and I was told my daughter would need to call since she was the last one mom spoke to. My daughter made the report. The person she was following never called the police, never called us either. It was my mom who called us and made us aware she was lost. My mother was lost for sixteen hours and found over fifty miles away. She was found early the next morning on the railroad tracks in Argyle, TX. When I called to thank the police officer for finding her, he stated, "something told me to go down that street, I never do." He saw the lights from the car on the track. He went to the car and opened the door. My mom told the officer she got lost going to a baseball game for my grandson. At this time the officer heard the train whistle blowing. He dispatched to the police department to stop the train. The train that day was held up while they removed my mother's car, it was stuck on the track. If not for this officer, and the whisper in his ear from God, I could have never made peace with my mother. I would have always questioned why she seemed to dislike me from 'out of the blue'…what a horrible thought.

It was at this time that I began the "beginning" of our journey, Mom's and mine. I hired an attorney, and realized many things were not the way she had wanted them. Mistruths were being told, and more importantly my mom was not being taken care of properly. She was a sick woman with a horrible disease. Pretending she was normal, did not make it so.

This was not an ordinary woman. She was the baby of eight children who was born to a poor family in Arkansas. She was married as a teenager, a mother by seventeen and a female police officer for the Dallas Police Department in her twenties. She would be a pioneer for all women in the 50's. A great mom, loving wife, devoted grandmother and great grandmother, loyal friend, and loving neighbor to all and everyone she met.

I knew it, church members told me, neighbors expressed concerns; the postal delivery person, Karen, pulled me aside with concerns. Now, I had to prove legally that I needed to be her guardian.

This was my mother and I would do whatever needed to be done.

It took a little over a year, but with the help of an intuitive court investigator and the Judge's findings, I was granted guardianship of my mom. We were able to bring in home health care. I believe this gave her extended life. In fact, I am sure of it.

In 2012 with the help of our attorney, APS, and caregivers findings, we were granted complete freedom for her legally. She was now a single woman who was free and was safe.

Due to this we were able to enter her home, I was shocked at the appearance of it. It clearly showed me just how sick she had become. The court had decided at that time to place her in a Memory Care Unit. I was her guardian, but they were still boss. I knew this was best. Now I took care of mom and of mom's home.

The saddest thing I saw in her house was a latch *outside* of the bedroom door with a combination lock on it.

One of the first questions she asked a care-worker when we placed her in memory care, "Are you going to lock me in here when you leave?" It was an arduous endeavor to bring my mother back into the realm of feeling safe and loved again.

Always listen to your inner voice, what friends and neighbors say. It is always good to have a professional to run things by. By the grace of God I was seeing a counselor who saw all the signs he had seen in his practice before. Talk to an attorney, a medical professional, get some help if you *doubt anything*! Unfortunately, there are those that prey on the mentally incompetent.

Someone Has To Take Over Where The Brain Leaves Off

I took my mom to her very first doctor's appointment before she got deep into her Alzheimer's. Even early on, she wanted me to fill out forms at the doctor's office. Many of the answers I did not know and she had to tell me. This was good because I needed to learn these answers. At the time, I did not know I would be filling out all of her forms in the future when she could not remember any of the answers.

Many years later, as per the first visit, it would be she and I going to see the doctor. The person who could have been taking her to the doctor seemed to have little concern for these matters. He had no problem telling me or a professional who asked, that he had no time to be involved in the care of Mom.

Mom and I went to many doctor visits and when she would be asked questions. It got to the point where Mom would just look over at me as if to ask, "What is the answer?" Most of the time I answered and the times I was instructed not to by a physician, I felt so guilty. I felt as though I was leaving Mom alone to fend for herself. Mom looked lost and quite sad because she did not have the answer and knew she should know it.

My mom was one of those people who could fool many people for quite some time. Socially she was like a butterfly. She could flutter here and there and smile and carry on a conversation. Occasionally, she would have a slip up and say something strange like she was going to buy you a house or someone had been in her home last night. Most people were not use to Mom having these slip ups so they excused her.

You will find that you, or someone close to your Alzheimer's loved one, will take on the role of their memory.

I learned more about my mom while I was losing her than I ever knew about her while she was well and in her right mind. While going through her things, after I got guardianship, I found a scrapbook she had. I had never seen this before. It was full of letters from different police chiefs at the DPD over the years. Each one praising her for a job well done. I found letters from individual citizens in the Dallas area complimenting her on helping to find their lost children. I found letters from companies, banks and other entities stating how she had helped to save their companies from a loss due to her police work. I found newspaper clippings and pictures. I just sat there and cried. I was in actual awe of this woman who was a hero and also my mom. A farm girl from Arkansas who came to the big city of Dallas, Texas with a two-month-old baby and a husband. She never had a job, and yet she talked my dad into letting her catch a bus so she could find her first job. She found a job on that first day, and started working at Singer Sewing Machine. Her next job would be the very first female dispatcher at the Dallas Police Department, and then on to the next venture as one of 17 women trying out for policewoman at the DPD. She would be the fifth policewoman hired to Dallas, Texas, badge # 2071. She was number two thousand seventy one, hired to the department in 1957.

The day I found all this information I realized, she can barely remember who I am. She does not know what day it is and most times cannot remember where she is or how to swallow her pills. I have become her memory. I have become her caregiver, the mom, the teacher and all things to her.

I realize all this and in that moment I am still in awe of her.

I found things my mom had written. Is this where my love for writing had come from? I never knew my mom wrote also. I found pages upon pages of records she kept. She made it very clear how she wanted things to be when she passed. I found what she wanted us to do with her belongings, her Will, her furniture, and her finances. My mom and Murray Katzen, her beloved and deceased husband she lost in 2000 saved everything. There were no doubts as to what they wanted, none.

My mother was so free from the influence of others. She was the most independent woman I have ever met in my entire life. In the end she was totally dependent on me. I was her memory. I was her defender. I was her advocate. I was her anger, I was her bodyguard, and I was her rock. Most of all, I was her daughter. I write about her for selfish reasons. My mom would never have spoken to anyone about her attributes, her accomplishments, her awards. I was her memory, and I would be her voice with my words. She was and is a legend for all women who are in the workplace today.

My mom would be the last child born to Rosa and she would witness the brunt of her mother's illness as well. This plagued my mom most of her life. It was her greatest fear that she would succumb to it too. She was poor and quite alone at times in a family where her mom spent many years tucked away in a mental institution back in the days where little was known about mental illness. My mom had very little mothering skills, except for those her older sisters taught her. I always knew she loved me and the last two years we had together were the best years of our lives loving one another. As I said, I found her while I was losing her and **I loved her all over again**, from beginning to end.

The Journey

JANUARY 12, 2010

Alzheimer's is like someone took your book of life and ripped out many of the pages, but those you love will never forget your story.

FEBRUARY 10, 2010

My Mom has been missing since 12:15 today. She has Alzheimer's and got lost while driving and following another car that belonged to the man she married in 2005. She called my daughter from a Shell gas station. She explained she got lost at a turn, could my daughter come and get her. She hung up when someone in the background asked why she was on their business phone. We have not heard from her in over 12 hours. If you live in the Dallas area, please look out for her and if not, please pray for her safety. A Silver Alert has been issued and WFAA.COM has issued an alert. My first questions was –WHY WAS SHE DRIVING?

From WFAA.COM

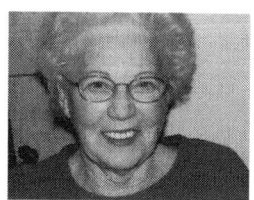
Silver Alert for missing Rowlett woman
ROWLETT — Rowlett police investigators have asked for the public's help to find an elderly woman. Rosemary Katzen, 75, was last seen in the 6500 block of Northwest Highway in Dallas, near Medallion Center.
Katzen was driving a 2009 white Toyota Camry sedan with Texas plates JRZ-491. Contact Rowlett police or your local police agency if you have any information.

FEBRUARY 11, 2010

"Rosemary Katzen was found safe early this morning in her car at an Argyle rail crossing" stated Rowlett spokeswoman Donna Huerta says.

My mother was found in Denton stuck on some railroad tracks and has been taken to the local hospital there. Thanks for all the prayers and thanks to the police officers that found her. Will let everyone know how she is doing later today.

"It is common for a person with dementia to wander and become lost; many repeatedly. In fact, over 60 percent of those with dementia will wander at some point." Alzheimer's Association.

FEBRUARY 20, 2010

"Too often we underestimate the power of a touch, a smile, a kind word, a listening ear, an honest compliment, or the smallest act of caring, all of which have the potential to turn a life around." -Leo Buscaglia

MARCH 2, 2010

Sending kudos to my daughter. I am VERY proud of her. Mindy, thanks for taking responsibility for a tough situation when it comes to a family member suffering from a terrible disease. I know this was one of the harder things you have had to ever work through. I love being a Mom!

MAY 25, 2010

"There is hope if people will begin to awaken that spiritual part of themselves, that heartfelt knowledge that we are caretakers of this planet." -Anonymous

JUNE 21, 2010

Alzheimer's can make you grateful...
Many times I take for granted
the simple things in life
The ability to remember an appointment
or even the date and time

I can wake up and know where I am
Go to sleep and know whose bed I am in
I am not constantly confused

And 'scared to death' from within

I don't put notes on my door
that read "no valuables inside"
I don't hear truths from loved ones
But, think I am hearing lies

I remember everyone's birthday
I remember my own past
I remember who hugged me
yesterday, and today…
who kissed me last.

I know where my keys are
I can find my own purse
I don't feel all confused
afraid, scared and hurt

I know someone who
was so independent
She was the strongest person
You could ever meet

And a terrible, terrible disease
has taken her away from me

I can still remember all and everything
I glimpse; a little of HER "aware"
Other times it is just the disease
I know SHE is not there...

Alzheimer's has taken
the best parts of her
But I will fill in the blanks,
fix any blurs
She would do the same for me
Mothers and daughters
are just made that way

JULY 19, 2010
Fading light...

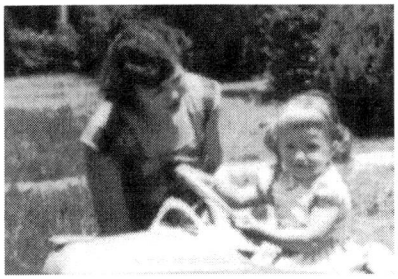

I know you are still there
Somewhere, yes somewhere
You will remember me
I will never forget you
A child never forgets
A mother's embrace
A kiss on the face
A bandage on the knee
The times you took up for me.

I ALWAYS thought of you as beautiful
To me you look just like you did then
The yesterdays, a child holds close within

In my sleep, I imagine you -
Brushing, my hair
Letting me sleep close,
When I was scared
As a child, so proud of her Mom
Because of her beauty in many ways
It seemed to make me feel
A little ok then -and now today

Or maybe I will never measure up
Or maybe I never can (in my head)
Or maybe I already have
 A little girl never forgets her Mommy

When she becomes a woman
She becomes a Mommy too
And the Mommy in me is part
Of the Mommy that was YOU.

I miss you Mom.
To all those out there who love or have a loved one with Alzheimer's, this poem is for you too. Xoxo

DECEMBER 21, 2010
Christmas memories past...

Will the real Santa please stand up?
Certain memories always stay with us, especially when it comes to Christmas. This is one I will never forget. It says so much about my mom, a little about old time beliefs and even more about what Christmas is all about. Love, love, and more love.

I am not quite sure what age I was, but an age that was still a very firm believer in Santa Claus.

It was Christmas Eve and I awoke to find I was alone in our home. Being that it was Christmas Eve, I knew the rules. You don't let Santa find you awake and here I was wide-awake on Christmas Eve. If I was not careful *he* might see me and I would not get anything for Christmas. I walked slowly through the house, room by room. No one was home. I slowly opened the door to the back yard. The whole time I was reminding myself not to look up into the sky. Santa might see me. I also vaguely remember wanting to call my mom's name but I was so afraid Santa would hear me.

I could not imagine what happened to my mom and dad, I had to find them. I decided to go to Peggy's house next door, my babysitter whom I adored. As I knocked on her door I was still hoping Santa did not see nor hear me. Peggy came to the door and as soon as she saw me she said, "Hi Honey." Peggy showed me unconditional love for many of my school-aged years. She invited me in and they had a house full of guests, my mom and dad being just a part of the mix. My mom came over to me and took me to the extra bedroom. I remember being tucked in and forcing myself to go back to sleep. I was still in fear of Santa finding out that I was awake.
I don't know how much later my mom woke me up but she asked me to go next door

and get her cigarettes. I put on my coat and walked next door to retrieve them for her. She said they were in the living area. At that time no one locked their doors at night. I walked into the house and then into living room. What did I see? I saw all these presents under the tree. Santa had come! Now what do I do? I better keep my mouth shut, I am thinking to myself. I went back to Peggy's and handed my mom her cigarettes. I noticed everyone was staring at me and I just took off my coat and went back to bed. The next thing I know my mom was back in the room and telling me to put my coat back on. We are going back to the house; I supposedly got the wrong cigarettes!

As we walked back into the house my mom yelled, "Look, who came?" So, I ran to see my presents, that earlier I had tried to run from, out of fear. Santa may have still been in the room, after all. My mom got down on the floor with me and we played for hours with my different colors of clay.

This was my momma who had come from a huge family back in the 1930's. They were hard working farmers. Mom married my dad and came to Texas for a better life. She became a mother, police Dispatcher, later a policewoman. She worked and attended classes at El Centro College. The woman that thought she was so ordinary, had a 4.0 average. My mom was considered a front-runner, pioneer, and career woman, when most women just stayed home in those days and took care of hubby and children. My mom was a true beauty in those days and is still a lovely woman even today. Her job as a policewoman put her on three different shifts and our time together was priceless, since it was few and far between.

Today my Mom suffers from Alzheimer's.

Of all things I hold dear, the thing that is most precious is the memory of every Christmas Eve when my mom would wake me up and tell me Santa had come. She could not wait to see me getting presents. It was not much in those days, but it was the fact that she was always just as excited as I was when I opened what "Santa" gave me.

The last few years before she became ill, she still gave presents before Christmas. Yesterday I wrote her a letter because sometimes it is easier for her to remember if she can read it. I put this story in there for her. Sometimes she remembers more things that are in the past than the daily things.

I just needed her to know that I remembered what a wonderful Santa SHE always was to ME.

Merry Christmas Santa (Mom!)

~ 2011 ~

APRIL 22, 2011

Ever had one of those nights when you try to sleep but all you can think about is solving every problem in the world? Yep, I solved all my fears, world hunger, the next election, aphids on my roses, my Mom's disease, my granddaughter Kenady's cough, my chocolate addiction, Johnson grass in my yard, losing weight, etc. But, I left out the cure for dark circles under your eyes from lack of sleep. I will solve that one tonight!

APRIL 25, 2011

The Big Red Hat at Easter

We had to sit up pretty high in the balcony at the church yesterday, and we even got there early. As I looked out over the crowd, it looked like a normal day at church. In fact, I only saw one hat. A big, red one with an enormous feather. It was an AWESOME hat! I am sure no one could see the pastor for at least three rows behind "the hat". But, I could have stared at that hat for an hour anyway.

That beautiful hat mesmerized me. It soon took me back to memories of years ago when my mom made most of my clothes. I always knew when it was close to Easter because I could smell the fabric on my mom's sewing machine. She had one of those OLD Singer push pedal machines. I would hear that thing spinning and wondered if she and it were one day going to let loose and spin out of that closet she did her sewing in. Would they meet up with the mean witch in the sky from the Wizard of Oz? She could make the most beautiful clothes on that ancient machine for many years until she became ill.

Who needed a store bought dress with a petticoat if my mom could make any dress for special occasions. It was scratchy, it was big, it was noisy, but I felt like a Princess in it. I could sit there in the church or at a birthday party and be encircled in the aroma of my crispy, new blue, or pink fancy dress all day long.

So, next year, I will be the one wearing a big fancy hat. Hopefully, someone just like me will think back to days gone by when things were bigger, fancier and yell, "Hey, look at me!" I will wear it in remembrance of every Mom who took time to sew her daughter a dress, one that was weaved in love and many sweet memories.

I wish I had taken the time to tell my mom I loved the dresses she made for me, but like every little girl I am sure I just complained about how scratchy they were.

Now, my mom has Alzheimer's and I try and tell her every time I speak with her how much I love her and how much she means to me. In my heart I know she still hears me and understands.

Love has a way of never losing its memory.

May 4, 2011

An Arkansas country girl who grew up and moved to the big city and became one of Dallas' finest policewomen, and you "wonder" why I have so much moxie. I admired your tenacity and drive, my beautiful mother. Xoxo

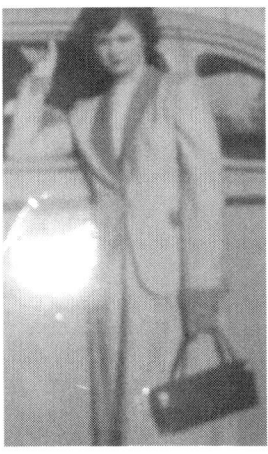

MAY 8, 2011

I love being a Mommy and I love my Mommy. To all the wonderful Mom's reading this, and to all the Moms who are in our hearts and memories, Happy Mother's Day today. Oh, and to all Mommy wannabes, it will happen, just you wait and see! xoxooxox

MAY 18, 2011

I adore my Aunt Dot. She is going on 80, and I asked her 4 days ago if she could get me two death certificates so I could prove to my mom that her parents were indeed deceased. Within four days, a 54 and 46-year-old document showed up in my mailbox. I can't even find a stamp in 4 days. Aunt Dot, I want to grow up and be as bright and on top of things as you ALWAYS are. I love you. xoxo

JUNE 3, 2011

I am finally winding down with one more EXTREMELY LONG task I have to finish. The last two years have been very tough on me due to my Mom's illness, but life goes on. I have a long-standing joke with an attorney friend of mine. We always joke and say, "I see the light at the end of the bar." Have a great weekend everyone and tell a blonde joke. Those are so funny! <Smoochies> xoxoo

JUNE 4, 2011

Drama, drama, drama! Thanks for your help tonight, Mindy. TOGETHER we can get through this process. You were my champion tonight. I love you! xoxo

JULY 30, 2011

I saw my Mommy yesterday for the first time in a few months. Long and sad story, but it was so good to see her. Of all things, I forgot my camera and we took pictures from a cell phone. The pictures are horrible quality, but you can still see her smile, and you can see our smiles. So if you focus on the smiles, it is a great picture.

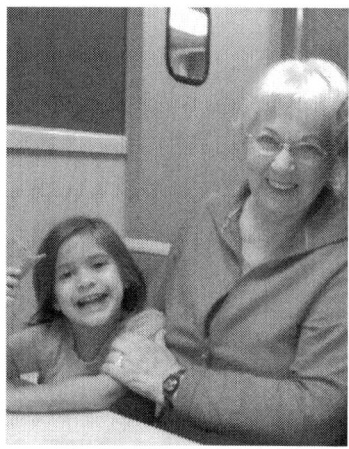

JULY 30, 2011

Wow, I can sure see God working in my life. I had a great visit with my Mom today. I also ran into some old friends who are so good for my spiritual well-being. I told you that shooting star last night was a message of love from God to ME. See, I am not crazy. I am happy today, and hopeful for my future and for those I love! xoxox

JULY 31, 2011

Wow, more insight and more understanding of what is going on in my life. We all go through trials and it just strengthens us and gives us an understanding of what others may want to take from us... God gave me a gift of joy and I am a joyful person! No matter what happens, no one can take that joy away from me. Good and God always prevails!

AUGUST 3, 2011

I just received wonderful news. The date has been set. August 22nd. Only a few more weeks, and we will have an answer for this journey that is taken over a year. I have learned so much over the last year about myself, professionals, neighbors, the legal system, home health care, FB friends, etc. I never have to be alone in any crisis. xoo-xoxo Let's find a cure for AD! xoxo

AUGUST 6, 2011

This is a picture of my Mommy holding my baby girl who turns...today. A woman never tells her age or her weight. This picture makes me smile as I am reminded what a gift she was the day she was born. Since then it has been another story. I am just kidding! I love her and I am going to kiss her all over, later today. xoxo

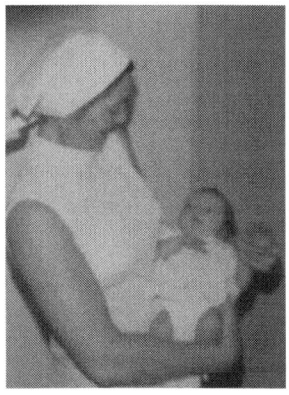

AUGUST 7, 2011

For a while I admit I was becoming a little cynical about the world and people in it, due to events going on in my life. But, God has given me the opportunity to see that He has always been here for me! I have been surrounded by an awesome network of people ready to guide me, love me and lead me. He had it all planned. Oh me of little faith. Today, I am sending kisses to my Heavenly Father. xoxo

AUGUST 10, 2011

When Alzheimer's affects a loved one, it makes some days harder than others. Today is one of those tough days. Tomorrow, I am sure it will be better. Happy Hump Day everyone! Sending out some love. xoxoox

AUGUST 13, 2011

Suzy Pitts-Smith, thank you so much for all of your help these last weeks, you and Dell both. When I was growing up, I always felt that the Dallas Police Department was like an extended family to me. I guess things never change when it comes to love and loyalty. I can't wait to hear from Mom's old friends and work buddies. It makes me feel like she is still "engaged" in a way. xoxoo

AUGUST 15, 2011

I am having so much fun talking to police officers my mommy worked with. They are all heroes to me, then and now. I love a man or woman in a uniform, even if it is just hanging in the closet. xoxoxoox

AUGUST 16, 2011

I wish my status line gave me enough room to put everyone's name that has helped me through this last stretch. I never knew how much my mom was loved, or how much love one will be given if only he or she asks. *"A single arrow is easily broken, but not ten in a bundle."* -Japanese proverb. xoxo

AUGUST 17, 2011

I will be glad when midnight gets here so it will be a new day. Today was a tough one for me, even with all my extended love and strength. I am sending out love to others who may need an extra source of hugs and kisses. xoxoxoox
Say to those with fearful hearts:
"Be strong, do not fear; your God will come, he will come with vengeance; with divine retribution he will come to save you."-Isaiah 35:4

AUGUST 22, 2011

God is so good! I am now the guardian over my mother. I have saved my mom. Mommy, I did it! All this hard work, all these long months, investigations, courtroom drama, phone calls, and records galore! All the love and encouragement from so many has paid off. Thanks to an awesome attorney and an awesome God! xoxoox

AUGUST 27, 2011 AT 1:56AM

The fading Star… (My Mom and her Alzheimer's)
I am starting a blog about my mom and how we are coping with Alzheimer's. I am

going to include colleagues she worked with at the Dallas Police Department, friends and family. It will primarily be about a daughter and her mommy. I think this is part of my "grieving process," as my lovely daughter, Mindy, said to me the other day. My mom was diagnosed after October of 2009. I have worked long and hard to get guardianship of her, and now, quite honestly, since getting it I am scared to death. The roles of a lifetime have been reversed and this is one of the biggest tasks I have ever taken on. I lose a little bit of her every day. I think it was Nancy Reagan who described the disease of Alzheimer's as the "long goodbye."

It is even worse when it happens to a woman that was the epitome of independence, sassiness and so full of life. Here I am an only child, trying to cope with the sickening, empty feeling that I cannot seem to shake. I go to bed with it and I wake up with it. The conscious knowing that she is leaving me and I don't know what I will do without her. I love to write, and I am hoping whatever I write about will help me, and maybe in some way, help other mothers and daughters. One of the things I have learned about this disease is that although my mom is still alive, we cannot connect. I can't say to her that I wished we had not argued about silly things. I can't tell her that I need her when I am down. I can't talk about when we last did something together.

Another thing I have learned is that friends are an awesome commodity in life, but a mom is your past. She is your time before, from the very beginning, and most likely she was the best mother she could be. My mother was not perfect, by any means. I was not the perfect mother to my own daughter. Just ask her! :)
Love is never perfect. It is forgiving. Regret is non-refunding.

SEPTEMBER 6, 2011
My hope was that today I would have some movement as far as my mom goes, but it looks like the Judges are all out of town until Monday of next week. Yet again, I play this waiting game. The judicial system is what it is. God grant me the serenity to accept the things I cannot change. The courage to change the things I can, and the wisdom to know the difference. Sending out love.

SEPTEMBER 19, 2011
I must have slept standing on my head...when I woke up my neck was stiff as a board and I am moving like Frankenstein. I need a good massage. This is going to be a busy week. I hope to get some things taken care of with Mom. Wishing all my Facebook buddies an awesome Monday. Sending some love your way. xoxo

SEPTEMBER 20, 2011

Most of you know Alzheimer's has become an integral part of my life. You watch your loved one deteriorate a little more every day, and you are helpless to stop the progression of the disease. My prayer is that more and more people will get involved so we can eradicate this horrible disease.

SEPTEMBER 23, 2011

"Holding on to anger is like grasping a hot coal with the intent of throwing it at someone else; you are the one who gets burned".- Buddha

I am trying not to get burned here, but sometimes it is tough when someone you love is involved. Acceptance is the answer to all of my problems today. That does not mean I have to like it, I just have to accept it for now.

OCTOBER 12, 2011

I spent the day with my mom and my big baby girl. My Mom was "engaged" today, and we laughed and enjoyed one another. I was able to get some of her medical needs taken care of and some of my "needing some mommy time" fulfilled. I know these days are few and far between, but with the disease of Alzheimer's, I will take whatever it spoon feeds me. xoxoox

OCTOBER 17, 2011

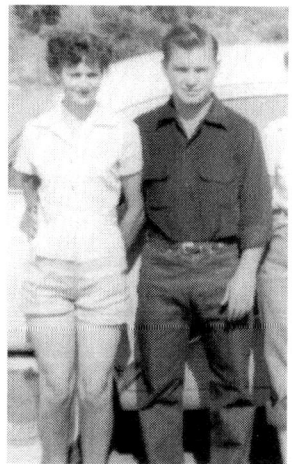

Some nights are harder than others when it comes to missing my mom. She holds all of my memories inside of her and only she has the key to share them. My dad, bless his heart, does his best to remember what I need, when I need it. But, Mom's and daughters have a special bond, even if we get on each other's nerves at times. When I was at Mom's the other day, I was able to get her book of old pictures. I remember as a young girl going through these all the time. These pictures are priceless to me. They are the reflection of who I was, and how my parents were absolutely the "real" Barbie and Ken. Hope you enjoy sharing my memories. xoxo

OCTOBER 19, 2011
About Mom and Alzheimer's (The missing shoes)

The Inventory

We have to do an inventory of the things in Mom's house for the court. It is such a long process when you get awarded guardianship. My daughter and I are working together on this very diligently. We are like the Three Musketeers, Mom, Mindy and "ME"; the three M's.

My Mom has this idea that someone is taking one shoe from every pair that she owns. I don't argue with her. To her it is the truth just like to me, I am sure I have to take a breath or I will die. In her mind this is happening. At the moment, it is her sister taking her shoes; tomorrow it could be Mindy or me. I am learning so much about this debilitating disease.

I told her I would help her find all of her shoes. I found some in the bathroom cabinet, some under the bed, and some under the couch. They were everywhere. My mother loved shoes. I found all the matches to about 40 pairs. She was so proud of me.

The sad thing is that these shoes looked so old and worn. I looked at the shoes she was wearing. They were a pair of lime green flip-flops. She needed a pedicure, and why was my mother wearing a pair of worn out, lime green, flip-flops? *I will take her shopping*, I told myself. It was obvious that she had been forgotten. Just like her shoes had been misplaced she had been lost too, in this horrible disease.

She is under my obligation now and I intend to buy her lots of new shoes and, of course, I will help her find each and every one that disappears and she will be proud of me every time. :)

No one's to blame
So much has changed
Though her beautiful smile

Remains the same

OCTOBER 20, 2011

I am bombarded with more papers that I need to go through so it's back to business as usual tomorrow. I think I live at my computer these days. I wish I had a nickel for every paper I have copied fifty different times. I have enough hell managing my own life, much less managing someone else's. But, I am alive, I don't have cancer, I can breathe, I can sing, although it's usually off key. I still have all my teeth, well almost, and I still have my joy. I have a lot to be grateful for. Acceptance is the key to all of my problems today. xoxooxox

NOVEMBER 2, 2011

Tomorrow is a big day in the saga of my mom's future with this lovely thing we call Alzheimer's. It will decide whether or not she gets her meds as directed and I can honestly be her guardian, or if we just keep playing this game of, "hurry up and wait and see." I am becoming a pessimist and I don't like that aspect of me. I don't know how many tests, how many doctors, how many written reports, how many times you need to go to court to prove a fact a five-year-old could figure out on their own. It gets a little depressing after a while. Protecting those that can't protect themselves is a thankless job, and a weary one to say the least. My thanks will come when she is in a safe place and professionals are finally addressing her needs! I still think we have the best judicial system in the world, but it needs some tweaking here and there, especially when it comes to the elderly and the mentally ill. I will never stop fighting for you, Mom! xoxoxo

NOVEMBER 4, 2011

I am dealing with an imbecile. I think God puts one of those in everyone's life. I have decided to make it a laughter thing. Instead of letting "it" get to me, I will make a joke out of this person's actions. My daughter and I will go forward and go by all of the rules. Everyone knows this person's true motivation. You can fool some of the people some of the time, but, well, you know the rest. Anyone want to sit in a hot *tube*? (An inside joke) with Shannon at the law firm. LMBO. I am sending out some love and I am not going to be a hater!

NOVEMBER 13, 2011

I finally got control of my mom's meds. It took me hours to decipher what was what, and I have ten years of experience working with medications. The generic brands are so confusing, and when someone hands you a container and pills that have been handled all willy-nilly, it is a nightmare to get them sorted. I got out my old physicians reference, used my computer, and finally figured out what was what. I think my mom may have been getting one or two of the right pills out of eight per day. No wonder all of her blood test results were horrible! There is absolutely no telling how much better she may feel now that she is getting her correct dosage, and the correct pills. I can see why there is such a fear is this country about getting older. This really concerns me for the elderly who are alone and have to take their own medicine.

NOVEMBER 16, 2011

I got my mom some "in home" health care today. They will start on Friday. I have a new book on Alzheimer's to read, and another person I can trust to assist my mom. Got the meds straightened out, called the pharmacy, called two doctors back, talked to my Dad, picked up a lock box with Mindy, went grocery shopping for my own groceries, and then had Sushi. You know the strange thing is, I did a lot of laughing today. I feel like I am getting some of the joy back in my life, or maybe it is just sheer exhaustion, who knows? I love being with my daughter. She is a good kid and it makes me feel like I accomplished one really great thing in my life, HER! I love you Mindy.

NOVEMBER 18, 2011

Wow, what a day! I spent time with Mom, met her caregiver and was highly impressed. The three of us met and had coffee after spending time with Mom. My mother may actually have a life now outside of her four walls. I may even have a life now without constantly worrying about my mom. To all her police buddies out there, call me if you want to see her. The caregiver can meet you, and you can spend some time with Mom. Mom was in a pretty good mood today and was even talking about some of her past work history. She would look at me if she forgot something. I love being able to remember the history she can't, it lets me fill in those empty spots for her. I think it makes her feel safer and isn't that what life is all about? Everyone needs a safe harbor, a soft spot to fall on, a puppy kiss, a human kiss and of course some chocolate. xoxoox

NOVEMBER 25, 2011

JOY, JOY, JOY! I had an awesome Thanksgiving. I was able to spend time with almost all of those that I love the most. My mom did really well yesterday; she laughed and was well engaged. I guess it helps when you get your medicine. My daughter made an absolutely wonderful meal. My grandbabies were our entertainment and The Cowboys won! Tomorrow, I will have about 17 people here. So, today I am doing my Christmas decorating. Next week, I will start my New Year's Eve decorations. Just kidding! I hope everyone had an awesome turkey day. Now we can work on losing those extra three pounds we gained. xoxoox

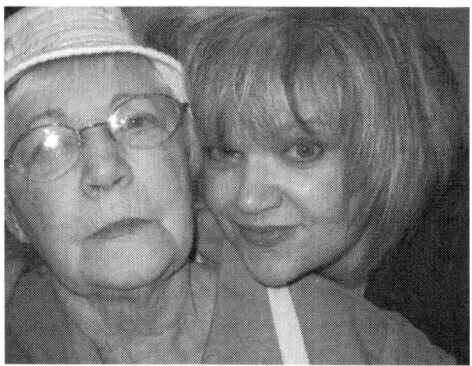

NOVEMBER 30, 2011

Patience, OH MY GAWD, give me patience today. I want to be angry, but I won't. I want to scream, but I won't. I want to kick the furniture, but I won't. I want to throw a toddler fit, but I won't. I will just know that some people are going to be who they are, regardless. I am the only one who can give them the power to hurt me or cause me to be angry. So, I will put my doll away and the four inch pins. Just kidding! Happy hump day to all of you lovely people. xooxo

DECEMBER 3, 2011

Thanks to all the "angels" out there who called my mom today. One of my dearest friends called her, and Mom said, "Well, I am having the best time. I have a big birth-day cake here and all my friends!" I am sure that is what she thought, with all the phone calls from old working buddies, old friends, family members, and my friends she knew. We will actually see her tomorrow for her birthday, but I wanted today to be special for her. Because of the wonderful people in my life and in my mom's life, she had that big birthday cake with all her friends "there." I have some awesome people in my life and an awesome God who put those "angels" in my mom's life today. xoxoxo Happy Birthday Mom!

DECEMBER 6, 2011

We took some pictures last night at dinner, but we decided to take crazy pictures just for fun for Mom. Her smile was priceless. Here we are in our "redneck Texas" pose. We may make this our Christmas pose this year.

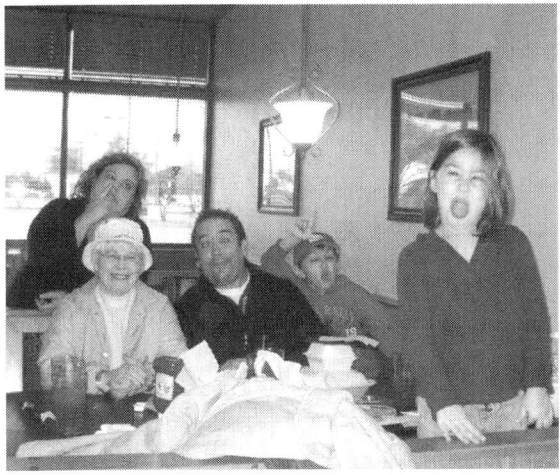

DECEMBER 12, 2011

I am reading a great book called "People of the Lie." It talks about the psychology of evil in the world, and in people. There can be a state of soul against which love itself is powerless because it has hardened itself against love. Hell is essentially a state of being which we fashion for ourselves; a state of final separateness from God, which is the result, not of God's repudiation of man, but of man's repudiation of God. This book has totally answered so many of my questions about why I get certain feelings around particular individuals, or things I see or read. Even with my rose colored glasses I have to admit there truly is evil in our world. I have faced some of it the last year and a half. This does not make me sad though. This gives me hope that we, as individuals, can fight any evil and face it head on whether it is in our neighborhood, in our government, in our extended families or maybe even in ourselves. God can, will, and does save us from any and everything we ask for. It is all a learning experience and I am learning.

DECEMBER 12, 2011
Whimsical version of a poem in my head tonight about mothers and daughters... :)

Mudders and dauders :)
Mothers and daughters
Oh, mudders and dauders
Sometimes best friends
Other times more cooler than hotter.
You look at them
It's like lookin' in a mirror

There's nothin' in your heart you hold dearer
But there are times you do want to scream
You do wonder "Why?" she just don't understand me!
Although questions arise,
The love is never denied.
As you get older you have regrets
About your own mother regrets with your own daughter
Like I said, sometimes more cool than hotter.
But, mudder's and dauder's should get along, Yep, they otter! :)

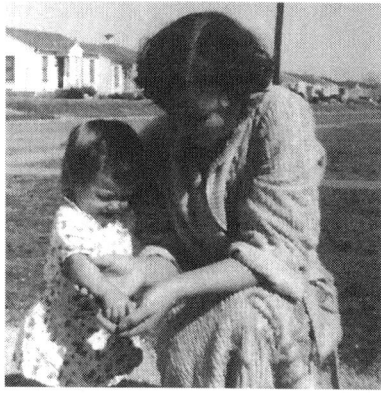

DECEMBER 13, 2011

Lunch was so awesome today. Alzheimer's causes so many different personalities in the person who is suffering. In the beginning, my mother said some awful and hurtful things to Mindy and I. I was wondering if we could ever repair the hurtful things that had been said to us. Since getting guardianship, getting her meds straightened out, and being more "in control" of her life, I have seen the gentle, kind, mother of mine awaken. Today, she would look at me and say, "You are so pretty," "I love you," "You are such a good daughter." At one point I reached over and rubbed her back and then her arm. It felt so good to touch her again. I kept telling her what a good mom she had been and then she told me what a good daughter I had been. I began to cry and she reached over to me and spoke to me like she did when I was a child. She said, "Don't cry little girl, I love you." I realized today that the best part of my mom is still inside her. I thank God for days like today. Xoxo

Christmas 2011, with Mom

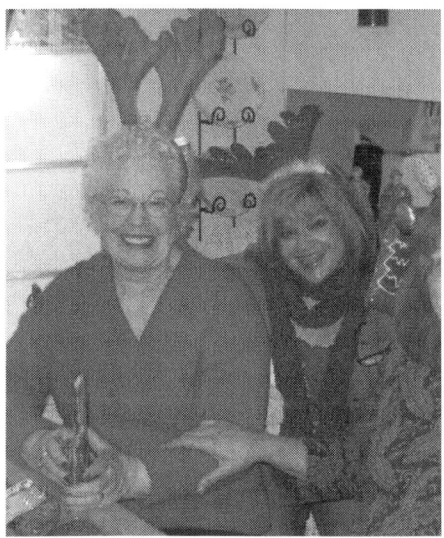

FEBRUARY 14, 2012

It is a good day. Things are getting settled for my mom. She has some awesome care-givers. I will swim tonight. I have some chocolate. It is a day of love and the sun was shining all day. This is one of those days I would like to bottle. Every day is such a gift from God. Some days feel like a gag gift, but it is still a gift. xooxox

FEBRUARY 24, 2012

It went well with Mom today. The Neuropsychiatrist says she is improving. Funny how that works when you get your meds on a regular basis. The agency we are using has been a real Godsend. Thanks Patsy! Now that I am home, I think I will take Pudge boy, my dog, and go to the park for a walk. It is a beautiful day here. I am learning to accept Mom's illness. I have no control over it, I can't cure her, and I did not cause it. It is kind of like everything else in my life. I just take it one day at a time. She smiled at me today and she knew who I was, and she asked me to pull up my jeans because she said she could see my butt. The X-ray eyes she now has are an added attraction, because I have NO idea how she could have seen my butt. Maybe she meant my lower back? Anyway, I love her and I accept her today and her Alzheimer's. xoxoxo Happy Friday everyone! Smoochies!

MARCH 15, 2012

Yesterday, my mom was more confused than usual. She asked Mindy who she was when she first arrived. I look at Mom, and while I am with her I feel as though I am able to handle it and things are "ok." When I am alone at night, after a visit with her, the sadness takes on a life of itself. I can tell she is regressing, or should I say, progressing, in her disease. It is at those times I get an emptiness in the pit of my stomach. The emptiness one feels when they have received a bad diagnosis from the doctor, or a call from a friend who is hurting. The feeling that comes with having question upon question in your head, and knowing there are absolutely no answers. It is a feeling of helplessness, loneliness and overwhelming sadness. I don't even have enough words to describe the concave that seems to engulf me at those times. It normally takes me days to get over my time with her when she is showing more signs of Alzheimer's. While I was there, I found two pictures of her I will post today. One was when she was 28 years old, and another in her Dallas Police uniform. My God, she was so beautiful and I miss her so much. It is times like this that I wish I could call her and tell her how sad I am feeling. God bless all the moms we miss and love. xoxoox

APRIL 3, 2012

Mindy, the caregiver, and Mom were having a great lunch today. I got a call from Tony about the storm coming our way. I grabbed Mom's roses, her muffins I made, and we loaded her up in the car. We all went our separate ways. I was sure I was going "away" from the storm. As I drove home, the rain was so hard I could hardly see and then it started hailing. I thought I was going to wet my pants I was so scared. I tried to find cover, but everyone was parked under all the carports at service stations. I crossed the street and found a drive thru for picking up prescriptions as I heard POUND, POUND, and POUND! I waited it out there, and then drove home. I noticed I was actually shaking. Mindy called me just about that time and said there was a tornado in Mesquite, five minutes from where I was going. That is just like me! Trouble doesn't follow me, I seem to run right into it!" This has been a scary day. Hope all my Texas buddies are safe and sound. xooxox

APRIL 4, 2012

Wow, I awoke to so many messages on my phone, and so many emails asking if I was ok and if my family made it through the storm yesterday. I felt so much pure love. I met a new caregiver for my Mom today, and now I have two that I believe are going to be real gifts from God. When saying "goodbye" to my Mom yesterday, she hugged me while we were standing and she rocked me back and forth. She would not let go of me. She whispered in my ear how much she loved me and that she wanted me to come and see her. To her, this was the first time "in her mind" she had seen me in a long time, although it was only days ago. I came home and called my dad who has been divorced from Mom for years. I could tell he was tearing up. Alzheimer's cannot stop love, years of absence do not forget love, and love is truly blind in all aspects of life. Thank you God for sweet, sweet love. xoxo

APRIL 7, 2012
Mom and Easter 2012

Mom continues to progress in her disease and has now started putting on more weight; my mother, who always had the perfect body. The perfect breasts, small waist, and a size 8 all rolled up into one gorgeous woman. She is, for the first time in her life, larger than me. These roles reversed seem so out of kilter. She still has the smooth, milky white, soft, skin. She still looks so young for her age, and she still has the humor everyone adores. She is still so beautiful.

I wanted her to look pretty for Easter. I looked through her closet on Thursday, and nothing seemed to really fit her anymore. So I went shopping. I found a beautiful suit that was very expensive. My mom would never buy something like this, she was so frugal. I could see her in it, she would look so classy. I also saw a blouse with lovely purple flowers; she loves purple so I decided to get it as well. I also purchased a nice pair of shoes. I wanted size 7 but the lady told me if she was a size wide she would need the 7 ½, so that is what I bought her.

I took the packages to her home. She asked me who I was. I smiled and said, "I am Mary, Mom." She said, "Where are your children?" I motioned for her to come to the bedroom. I told her I had surprises for her.

She tried on her clothes and everything fit but the shoes were flopping on her feet. She told me she would still wear them since I had bought them. I told her that was not feasible, she would fall in them. I could tell she felt bad that they did not fit, only because she was afraid it would hurt my feelings.

She began to tell me how much she loved some man who had come by in a truck with another man, and how she had wanted to chase the truck and jump in the back of it. How this man had been so handsome, and that when she saw him she thought he might leave her. She kept repeating how much she loved him. I was wondering if she was speaking of her deceased husband, Murray. She had a great love for him. This left me puzzled. I wanted to go home and call my dad. After we visited some more, I said my goodbyes and left.

When I got home, I called Dad and explained the story to him. At first he could not remember a truck. Then it dawned on him. He and his brother, Dayton, had a white truck and had picked Mom up in it. It was a long, funny story about how the drive shaft had fallen out of the truck and they lost control in the woods.

My dad began to tell me how he and Mom had a special love. A love like no other he had before. Of course, I began to cry like a baby. My dad still loves my mother, it is evident.

Every son or daughter, I imagine, wants to feel like they were born from pure, sweet love. I have often wondered where my capacity of love comes from. Since my parents divorced when I was 17, and divorces are never happy or amicable, we often forget the love our parents felt for one another.

One of the many things my mom's disease has actually given me as a gift is her past memories. I can relive her old memories. She takes me back to happier times she may never have shared with me due to old hurts. She takes me back to a time when she adored my father, and then he can share with me the deep, young love they experienced.

Forgiveness comes in all forms. I believe Mom and Dad are forgiving one another through me. I cherish being that vessel of their long lost love.

Easter is all about faith, hope and resurrection. In this case the resurrection of a love that had long seemed dead.

MAY 2, 2012
About a daughter facing her Mother's Alzheimer's

Every time I visit with my mother I see her digression. I visited with her again this week. Her disease has now progressed into bouts of paranoia and seeing things on her body that are not there. Of course, this breaks the core of my being. I left my daughter's house on Tuesday in tears. I feel like, at times, she and I cannot lean on each other because we both carry the brunt of most, or all, of the heartache concerning Mom. One thing I realized on Tuesday was that immediately after I walked out of Mindy's house I was hiding my tears. I left without even hugging my own daughter goodbye. I was trying to be strong. She sees me get so upset so often over my mom. There is no greater bond than the one between a mother and a daughter, a daughter and a father. These are our parents. The people we thought of as God like figures when we were young; no matter how many arguments we may have had. We still see our past, present and future when we look at them. Inside of them lies the little boy or girl we once were.

I sat in my car asking myself, as I often do, *why*? I felt such sadness for my mother. I kept thinking that if she knew what she was saying or doing, she would be so embarrassed. She would never want to be like this. I felt such empathy for her situation, her decline. The only saving grace concerning this disease is that she does not know.

At times like these, God always provides me with exactly what I need. At that very moment I got a text asking me how my day was going. I answered back and said, "Horrible." The answer back was fast, swift, and comforting. It contained a few words of encouragement and understanding. Later, I would speak with her caretaker and received more words of encouragement. Then I talked to my stepsister, who knows Mom almost as well as I do. When I came home I had an email from the owner of the agency who provides her caretakers. She and I have become friends; she even attended my birthday party in February. My cousin called me later that night and she gave me more love and hope. Tonight I received a message from a Facebook friend I have never even met in person, yet, her kindness was overwhelming.

At times I question God about the "Why's" of the disease. Why MY mom? My beautiful, energetic, witty mother. There is no answer except, Why not? We don't get to pick and choose what happens to us in this life.

I believe it is all a learning and loving experience. I have learned to love my mother more than I ever could have before. I have learned to appreciate my own life more. I have learned to appreciate my own mind and memory more.

God knows exactly what I need when I am in my pain base. I don't know anything but the pain of losing my mother on a daily basis. These are the times He has to carry me to the place where I need to be.

I hope at times I have been that text that phone call, or that comforter to those who have comforted me.

Much love for all those who are hurting, no matter what the cause may be. xoxoox

MAY 8, 2012

I saw my mom today. She wore red and she looked gorgeous. She seemed better now that she is on some different meds. An in-home nurse will assess her tomorrow for physical therapy, or other needs she may have. I have the most awesome caregiving agency. If anyone ever has an elderly loved one who needs care, just ask me who I use. Mom, you looked beautiful today, and I cherish every day I have with you.

MAY 9, 2012
Mommy, Mom, Mothers

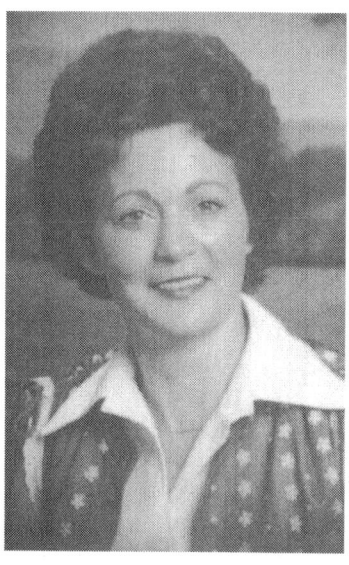

Happy Mother's day to all mothers
When you are conceived
Your mommy is your heartbeat
When you are an infant
Your mommy is your sweet retreat
When you are a toddler
Your mommy is your balance
When you are a preschooler
Your mommy is your teacher
When you are in Elementary
Your mommy is your idol
When you are in Middle School
Your mom is your rival

When you are in high school
You Mom is not as smart as you
When you go to college
Your mom's lessons you review
When you get married
Mom becomes the guidance counselor
When you have children
It's mom you call, because she's no amateur
When you get older
Your mother is your best friend
When your mom gets older
You are her lifeline till the end
It all comes full circle
A mother and a daughter
Always connected one
Way or another...
Till the end of time and beyond....for forever.
Dedicated to my Mom who suffers from Alzheimer's.

MAY 11, 2012

One of my Mom's favorite caregivers had to leave her position today. Her husband is very ill. Now we get to start all over again. I trust my agency, but sometimes in life I feel like it is two steps forward and one step back. But, at least I am going in the right direction.

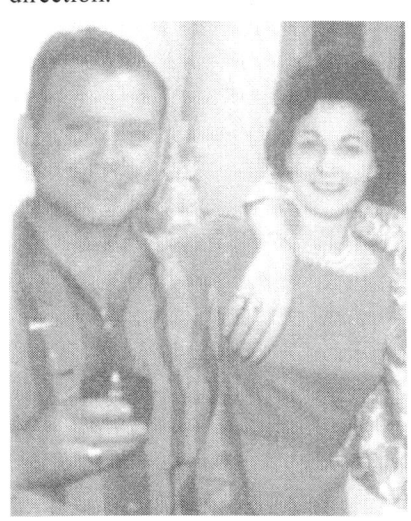

MAY 12, 2012

Mom and Dad when they were still together. I think I was about 14 when this was taken. They were Barbie and Ken, except Mom did not have blonde hair. But look at her body!

MAY 12, 2012

Happy Mother's Day to my beautiful mother, tomorrow, and to all the Mom's out there. Dad, thank you for still loving Mom even though you guys have been apart for many years now. If it was not for your continued love and support I would not have been able to get through another mother's day having Mom here but not having her "here." Mom, one day you will know.

MAY 13, 2012

Mother's Day

Even the dog got involved in this picture. As usual, Kenady is the star attraction. LOL

MAY 17, 2012

My mom had two great loves in her life. My dad, and the man she was married to until he passed in 2000. I just found out he is in a book about Rangers in World War ll. I looked him up online. He received so many medals during his service to our country. If they awarded a medal for being a "Mench" he would have received that medal in life.

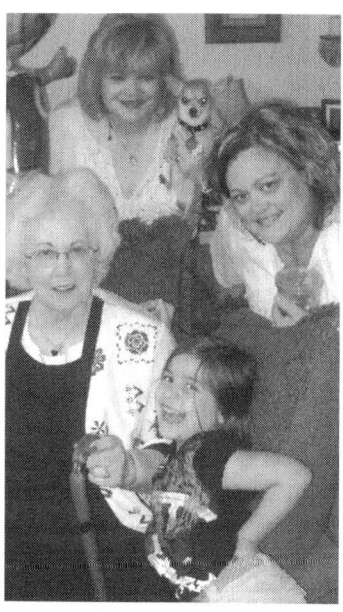

Sometimes, when I am alone with her she will look at me and say, "I have had a good life." The more I delve into her past, I would have to agree. Yes, Mom, you have definitely been loved by two wonderful men and been extremely adored by many. xoxo

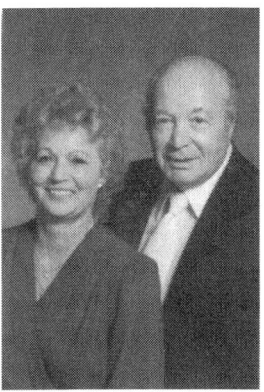

JUNE 16, 2012

Today was one of the scarier days of my life. My mom, caregiver, grandbabies, Mindy and I were all having lunch around 1:00. I looked over at Mom and she started falling over in her chair, my daughter caught her before her head hit the floor. She started seizing and we called 911. Mom, Caregiver and I immediately went to the doctor's office, because Mom would not go to the hospital. In the doctor's office she almost had the same episode. Needless to say, she and I ended up in the ER and now she is in the hospital. I just walked through the door almost 11 hours later. My mom and I bonded so much today. She was lucid more than not; she will have a lot of tests on her brain tomorrow. Mom, I wish you knew how you won over everyone at that hospital with your charm and beauty, even at 77. Patsy, Barbara, Judy, Mindy, Bradyn, my GAWD, I could NOT have gotten through this day without your love and support. Please send some prayers by way of my sweet mom. I will keep everyone posted. xoxo

JUNE 17, 2012

Quick update on my mom, they are still running tests. She is getting lots of attention from family and caregivers and nurses. I took her some Angel perfume tonight and she decided to spray it on Bradyn and me. Man, I am reeking right now, but in a good way. Love you Mom. xoox

JULY 3, 2012

Well, we will take Mom to the Cardiologist tomorrow. I am anxious to see what they have to say about the results of the tests done at the hospital. I am also afraid of what the findings are and of any new tests that will need to be done. Of course Mom will not understand, and for her that will be a blessing in disguise. I know in times like these I am never ever alone. Sending back some of the love I am always receiving. xoxoxoxo

JULY 5, 2012

Well, I had another funny adventure with Mom at the doctor's office. I did have a blog about the grandbabies but I may have to start one about Mom's "funny" quotes. An Alzheimer's patient always reverts back to many years in the past because they have such short-term memory, part and parcel of the disease. Mom has decided to start "playfully" hitting. Unfortunately, I am usually in the range of play. I think I am going to start sitting Mindy next to her. When they were doing the extensive tests on her heart she was giggling and laughing about how her heart sounded like an old washing machine she had right before it went Kapooie. When she was introduced to the doctor, who was young and cute, she said, "You sure are cute!" When I told her not to flirt she playfully hit me on the arm. OH LORD, I sat too close again! They sent her home with a 24hr heart monitor instead of a 30-day one. I can just imagine what she would have done to the electrodes in those 30 days! Anyway, we should get the results very soon. Mom is playful, giggly and still remembers who I am much of the time. So, today I am grateful for this and also for Patsy Corliss, owner and friend of my favorite caregiving agency. Patsy, I don't know what I would have done if you had not come into our lives and especially into Mom's. You are very special to me and you will always be. xoxoxo

JULY 10, 2012

I just found this pic of my mom (Rosemary Katzen), me and Mindy Michelle Stevens, the day she retired from the DPD after 32 yrs. This really takes me back. Yes, I was a chunky monkey in those days but let's focus on Mom, and how cute Mindy was and still is. Mom, I was, and still am, so proud of you. What would we do without pictures? Wow! Xoxoox

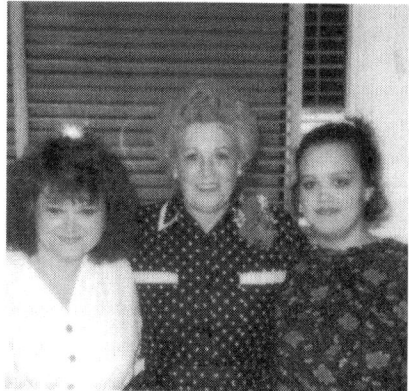

JULY 11, 2012

One of the major components in my life is to love and being loved. It comes in all shapes and sizes, all forms, male, female, animal, mineral and vegetable. Well, maybe I have gone a little too far. But, love is so vitally important to the human spirit. I received a card yesterday from someone I have only spoken with in short intervals throughout the years. We have discussed some of the things going on in my life with my Mom. She has one of the sweetest spirits and I have always been drawn to her. On the outside of my card she wrote "Mary" in all different colored squiggly letters. It was so cute and so personal. When I read the words in the card, I got really emotional. It included beautiful words of encouragement and a lunch invitation. I wonder sometimes what the world would be like without the love and thoughtfulness we receive from others on a daily basis. I am blessed to have so many friends I love, and they love me back. Here's to all the "earth bound" angels in my life. *Die Engel die mich umgeben sind der Schatz in meinem Leben*, Translation: The angels that surround me are the treasures in my life. P.S. I have to practice my German. xoxo

P.S. Thanks B.

JULY 23, 2012

What a day, what a day! Ambulance had to be called for Mom again today. This is right on the heels of Friday, when she had to go to the doctor for an infection in her toe, and had to be treated with antibiotics. Tomorrow we go back to the Cardiologist. The Neurologist is conferring with the Cardiologist to see why the recurring syncope. I went to her house to check on her today. I put lotion on her feet and legs, and curled her hair. She thought she looked beautiful and she did. How can you ever repay a mother?

Mom, thanks for all the hot meals you left in the oven for Dad and me when you worked the third shift. xoxoox

JULY 24, 2012 AT 4:39AM
Notes from the daughter of a mother with Alzheimer's
I cannot find my Mom
I look everywhere
Inside her brain
To find her, but the
Maze has defeated me.
I can still make her laugh
I love to hear her laugh

The really tough times
Are the times she looks
Straight at me and asks
Where's my Mary?
I look into her hazel eyes...
I smile and say, "I am right here"
She smiles back,
And says,
"I love you"

JULY 25, 2012

Update on Mom: She has to wear a heart monitor for 30 days, 24/7. This monitor has more parts than my IPhone. She does not understand why this apparatus is hanging around her neck. She requires more care now. Although I am her guardian, everything must be approved through the courts. Yesterday, within minutes, I actually had the doctor and the attorney speaking to one another. Mindy said, "In my entire life I NEVER expected to see such a feat accomplished." Mom kept asking why this thing was around her neck and blinking. I finally said, "Mom, UFO's may be trying to contact us and you have to be available to get any message they could send us at any time." She looked at me and started giggling like crazy. It eased her tension. More care means less tension for me and more safety for her. And who knows, maybe she will get some message from ET.

AUGUST 5, 2012

We are celebrating my baby girl's birthday today, although tomorrow is her actual birthday. Geeze! I cannot believe she is turning 25. I say this every year and will repeat it again next year, Mindy Michelle Stevens I carried you for 10 months, and I thought you were never going to be born! You have never been on time since then. See you later for sushi! By the way, I love you! Xoxo In this picture I think you were already about two weeks late.

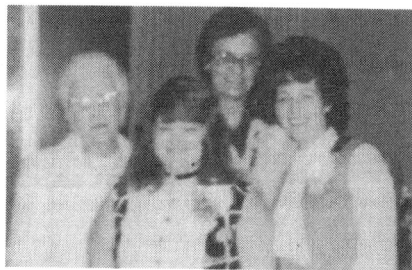

AUGUST 9, 2012

More drama today with my mama, and by no fault of hers. I think today had a little serendipity mixed in with it. God seems to put exactly the right people in my life just when I need them. Lately, He has been surrounding me with the most loving and kind people. I guess He knows what I need...hmm, He is funny about that! Even though it was a very stressful day, at one point it turned positive. It is due to friends, family, professionals, neighbors and God knowing exactly what I need and whom I need it from. God, let my hard times be healing times. xooxo

AUGUST 22, 2012

My daughter, my mother and a caregiver were at my house on Monday. My mother continues to progress in her disease. We have to make some serious decisions and many things are happening at the present time. I tend to make most decisions with my heart and my daughter is more prone to use her head. We even each other out, I suppose. Monday, as I looked at her freshly tanned face, I saw a little rash on her cheek, possibly from too much sun. At that very moment she reminded me of a little girl who came home from school one day, and asked me if she could give her bike to someone who had lost theirs. She was upset when I said, "No." So, under that tough exterior is still that little girl who is probably more like me than I realize. Family is so important! My daughter is helping me to live through "the daily loss" of my mother. I know some days I only think with my feelings. Thank you, to my daughter Mindy, for being there to even me out. I love you, Mom. X

xoxoox

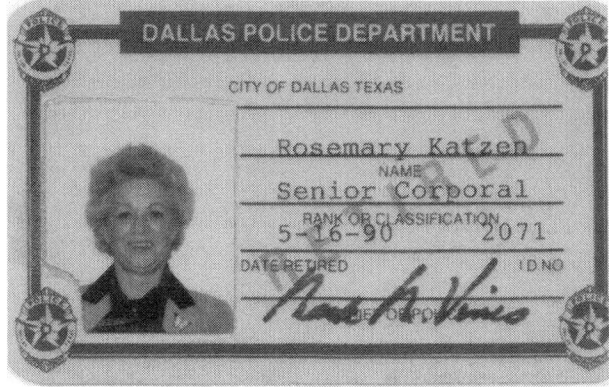

AUGUST 24, 2012

This whole journey was all about you, Mom. The victory is all yours. I wish you could awaken for five minutes so you could see just how many people were, and still are, in your corner each day. Mindy and I will never leave you. We will never stop loving you for who you are, for the lives you touched, and the way you continue to teach me things about myself each day. What an inspiration your life was and is. Your loving daughter, Mary.

AUGUST 29, 2012
...about a daughter who is living with her Mother's Alzheimer's

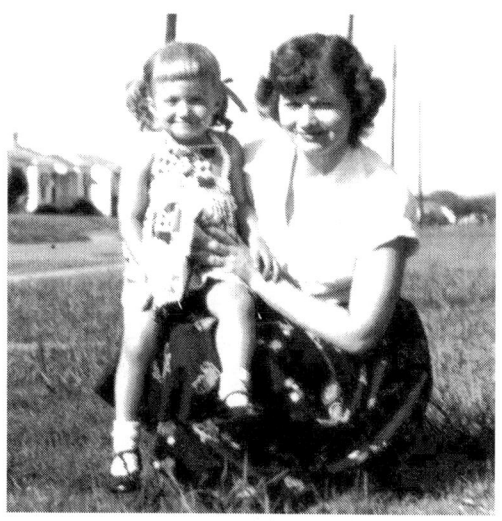

I love you more

I was with my mom tonight. Every time she sees me she stares at me with her beautiful hazel eyes and the first thing she says to me is, "You are so pretty." My mother was never one who gave out compliments easily. These days this seems to be the first thing she says to me. Her words are like warm, water flowing over my soul.

When I was young we never had much time together, she worked so many different shifts at the DPD. She also did part time work at James K. Wilson, in Wynnewood Shopping Center, as a "fake" customer watching for shoplifters. So, the little bit of time we had together was very valuable. We would always lie together on the couch and watch TV. I would be at one end and she at the other.

Tonight, she had a hard time going to sleep. I asked her if she wanted me to lie next to her. She smiled and said, "Yes." I climbed up in her bed and she moved over to give me room. She took my right arm and placed it over her heart, and then she kissed it. She hugged my arm and then looked up at me and said, "I love you," and kissed me. I

hugged her, cheek to cheek, and held back all my tears with as much strength as I could and said, "I love you more." I could feel her heartbeat as she dozed off.
Good night Momma...

SEPTEMBER 8, 2012
Living with my Mom's Alzheimer's
On Friday night, I was with my mom and a group of others who suffer from the same disease. I will use fictitious names to protect identities. Amy sat to the left of my mom, and was in a wheel chair. She had the most gorgeous, and stunning blue eyes. Her mind seemed to work like a prestigious, former schoolteacher. She was reading and did not skip a beat. She sat straight and tall, and she would tell people how lovely they were as they passed. Then there was my mom with her cane. She would playfully threaten to hit you over the head if you "messed" with her and then let out a laugh. She poked one woman in the backside playfully. The gentleman who sat next to my mom loved the attention he was getting, and though he said very little, his genuine smile gave him away. Mom offered to arm-wrestle him; he smiled and shook his head, no. As people passed the group, they would come in and say they wanted to join due to all the laughter. Laurie, the caregiver, and I laughed and laughed as all of these wonderful people acted like teenagers. Betty wore a key around her neck, and not once did I see her smile disappear. She would lean back in her chair and say she had never had so much fun! They acted just like my friends and I do! The only difference being, the next day we would remember what we had said and what had happened. But, they were happy at that moment. I heard their stories repeated many times over, but in all honesty I enjoyed hearing them time and time again.

This experience gave me a different outlook on Alzheimer's. There could be some joy found in the midst of the pain, the pain of seeing my mom lose her memory. Inside her was still that playfulness, that joy of being with others, the playful flirting and even being in a clique. The mind may lose its capacity to remember, but deep in the recesses of it still laid the most important things God placed there. The need for love and companionship no matter what we suffer from, never leaves us. I believe that love is not the last thing to go, I believe it never goes. You can silence love and you can take away its memory, but it still remains the most indomitable part of the human spirit. Thank you God for allowing me to see that NOTHING defeats love, not even Alzheimer's. xoxo I loved seeing you laugh and have fun, Mom. Xoxoox

SEPTEMBER 11, 2012

Just a little tribute to my wonderful, deceased stepfather, Murray Katzen: Murray was Jewish and my mother Christian, but they made it work. We celebrated Hanukkah and Christmas each year. I learned so much about the Jewish faith from him. We argued a lot about our differing views, but we each allowed the other to have them. In all reality they were not that much different. Murray taught me how to be tolerant of other people's beliefs. Who was I to judge another? Murray was kind, giving, and thoughtful, and treated my mother with an abundance of love. She had two great loves in her lifetime, my Dad and Murray. In the Yiddish language, being a Mench describes "a person of integrity," and that is surely what he was. I loved him for loving and caring for my mother, and I came to love Israel because he taught me so much about it. Such a little, tiny speck with so much hate around it. God bless Israel, and please keep her safe!

SEPTEMBER 13, 2012

When I get to Heaven, one of my first questions is going to be, "Why didn't I get my mom's long legs?" Then I will move upward to the rest of her body and finish with my questions. LOL Geeze, Mom! No wonder I always wanted to look just like you!

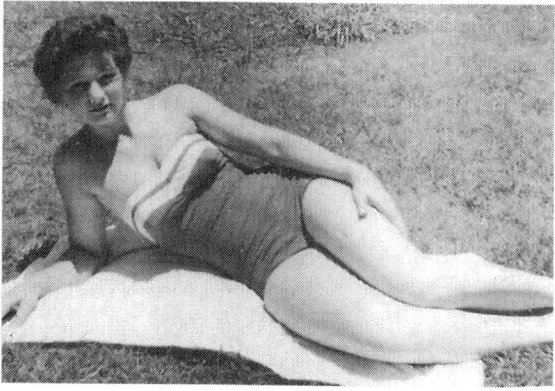

SEPTEMBER 21, 2012

Rocky Miele, it was so good to talk to you last night. You brought up wonderful old memories of Murray. You sounded just like he did when you repeated certain things he would say. Mom and Murray were blessed to have great friends like you and Lisa. She still has an old picture of you guys at a Christmas long ago. She adored Cleo. I hope one day soon you can come and see her, she may still remember you on a good day. Thanks again for being a great neighbor to her and to Murray. Much love

SEPTEMBER 25, 2012

As I walked in Mom's room tonight, she held out her arms really wide and said, "Where have you been, I have missed you so much!" and then she added, "Come here and give me a kiss!" Alzheimer's does have its rewards, they may be small, but it is the little things that you try to grasp on the bad days. xoxoox

OCTOBER 5, 2012

Mom, Mindy and I were scheduled to have lunch together today. Unfortunately, I was under the weather. Where did that saying come from anyway? Mindy sent me pictures. Of course, what do I do? Cry! Well, what do you expect? My two favorite girls enjoying being together and having their all-time favorite food, Mexican! I love you Mom and Mindy. Happy Friday everyone! xoxooox

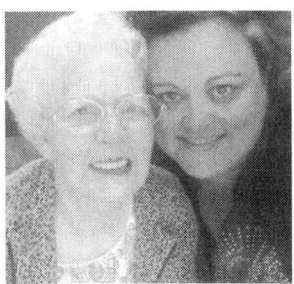

OCTOBER 10, 2012

The "enlightenment" of Alzheimer's disease

After being with my mom today, I noticed certain things when I got home.

1. My cat, Cashmere, has two front paws with black fur under the pad of the paw. The rest of her is tortoise shell color.
2. The hair on the back of my head is curlier than the rest of my hair.
3. The home I live in shifts every season, I can tell this by the way the doors gets tighter when you close them.

I started thinking; *I am noticing such silly, insignificant things for the first time yet they have always been there.* Well, maybe my hair is getting curlier as I get older. :)

But, I notice things more now. I am more in tune with my feelings, thoughts and emotions. Mom's disease, and all the other things along with it have changed me. In the beginning I was very angry and confused. I had questions such as; how could God take my mother away from me or why my mother?

Why not my mother? I am a firm believer that nothing in this life happens by chance. This is not to say I am not devastated by the prognosis, but I am gradually learning to accept it.

I met a wonderful man today; he prayed with me and gave me hope for the future. The disease gave me the opportunity to meet this man and share with him and let him comfort me. I also met, in person, someone I have been speaking with on the phone with. She was kind and loving and caring. The disease gave me the opportunity to make a new friend.

My mother is happy, she is safer than she has been in years, and she is loved. God did not take my mother away from me. He gave her back to me so that I could take care of her and love her the same way she cared for me for 18 years.

No matter what happens in our lives, we may never get the answers we want, but we will, and can, get the love and comfort we need from God and whomever He puts in our lives to help soften the blows.

Thank you God for insight today, even in the silly things in my life but especially in the big things. xoxox

OCTOBER 17, 2012

Do you ever just sit at the end of the day and reflect on how many people you have spoken to that day? How many people's lives are much like yours? How something they said related to your own life? Sometimes you will get a text, and it is a reminder that someone still cares about you. A call reminding you that you are still welcome to come over and carve a pumpkin; or just inquiring about how your day is going. Today, I bet I spoke with at least 25 people, some in person, some on the phone, some in text. A few were people who shared the same heartache I do with my own mother, as their mother or wife is going into Hospice. We all share a common cord, bond, and lifeline, whatever you would like to call it. But, it is all the same. We are different in race, creed, color, and religion, even politics. But, on one level we are all the same, we have all felt some type of pain in our lives and, God willing, we can be there to minister to others. Some are further along in their acceptance than me, and I let them 'carry' me when I am too tired. But, they give me "their" strength to go on. I hope I am always there to help others when they get too tired to go on. Thank you, God, for creating such marvelous, thoughtful, loving, human beings. xoxo

OCTOBER 24, 2012

...of a daughter who is dealing with her mother's Alzheimer's....

I really miss her tonight, daytime is easier for me. Tomorrow when the sun comes up, it will be better. It is nighttime that is the worst. I remember as a child being so afraid of the dark and she would let me sleep in bed beside her to comfort me.

Tomorrow when it is light, I know it will be easier.

If I had one wish, I wish I could call her and we talk about insignificant things. I wish I could "connect" with her just one more time. I would tell her how proud I am of her, how beautiful she is and was to me. How I always wanted to be 'just like her'... Just a short phone call, she would answer and I could say... "Hi Mom, what are you doing?" and she would ask me the same. We can still talk, my mom and me. But I no longer know the person who she is. I am so fearful of the day when she will no longer know who I am.

I love you Mom, sleep well, and sweet kisses for you.

Xoxooxo

OCTOBER 28, 2012

I hate you Alzheimer's

Today, I hate what you have done to my mom. She would hate you too. Everyone around her despises you. Today, I am drowning in fear and have many questions as to why. You have robbed me of my beautiful mother and of the time we could have together. She keeps asking me where her mom is, her father. They are both gone, many years ago. How am I supposed to answer this? I know the rules, I have learned the right answers to these questions, but it still does not make the pain stop when she asks me this. Does this mean she is going to die soon? Does she see them? Are they calling to her? Yes, these questions do invade my mind, and rob me of serenity. Isn't it enough that she is a mere shadow of who she once was? Today, I am angry with you, maybe tomorrow it will be easier; maybe tomorrow she will be better. Tomorrow, I may have more acceptance. Please God, give me acceptance and give my mom peace.

OCTOBER 29, 2012

Happy Halloween week everyone. I love all the pictures that are being posted. I am posting last year's pic, so I have a Halloween theme. I consider Halloween a big masquerade party, nothing more and nothing less. Mindy and I decorated cookies with Mom, and made a sugar cookie look like a pumpkin by putting orange icing on it and a green stem made out of icing. She loved it. Have a safe week BOOtiful people. xoxoox

OCTOBER 30, 2012
I had a dream of gardenias... (from the daughter of a mother with Alzheimer's)

Have you ever had a dream but did not remember it until you needed to? I had the most beautiful dream sometime in my sleep Sunday I was dealing with some pure, unadulterated anger today concerning Mom's disease. I was eventually driven to tears. I remembered the dream I had and immediately remembered how Mom and I had always sat on the porch at our home in Oak Cliff. Two huge gardenia bushes surrounded it, one on each side of the steps where we sat together. The smell of those flowers was heavenly. The dream I had was of an English garden that was covered in flowers but there was only one type of flower in the whole garden, and it was the gardenia. They were glistening and the dream was so peaceful. My dream, I believe, was from God, to give me solace for days like today, and to be able to remember the days my Mom and I sat together on the porch.

The dream
I dreamed of an English garden
It was full of beautiful blooms
The leaves were glistening and lush
As the dew was lightly touched;
by the morning sun.
All the petals were soft and round
Attached to thin long stems
The fragrance lightly sweet and so profound

An old wooden bench
Hidden in the corner
Surrounded by the bushes,
Almost hidden by the blooms

A peaceful encounter
A wonderful dream
I can close my eyes now
And smell its perfume.

One of those dreams

You do not want to awake
And want it to be real
Sorry to realize it was fake

So many dreams
These days are not these
Fanciful ones, but full of fear
And some, even hate

But in my dream of the Garden
It was of pure love and sweet memory
And for me
The gift of God's DIVINE GRACE.

NOVEMBER 5, 2012

My daughter and I are fighting the battle of our lives; we are fighting against Alzheimer's, which includes other "demons" right now. When I spoke to her a few minutes ago, she said she described us to someone today as "The Monster." She was the legs, arms, and body. I was the brains and heart. She said she thought we made an awesome team. My mother would probably totally agree. "The Monster" will fight for Mom/ Nana till the end! I see so much of my mom in Mindy; she is strong, resourceful and faithful. I am very proud of my daughter and I like the idea of us being a team, especially since she is my best friend too. I love you Mindy. xoxoxo

NOVEMBER 8, 2012

I am getting ready to go and see Mom with the kids and Mindy. I bought her a warm, fuzzy, purple top. She loves purple. I got her some sugar-free, chocolate candy and it looks yummy! (Slapping my hand) I also got her some fuzzy booties. I love the look she gets on her face when she sees us. One thing I am learning through the counseling concerning her illness is that she does not remember time as we know it. But, she knows when we are there even if she does not "know" like you and I do. Today, I am grateful she still knows who we are.

Hope springs eternal in the human breast:
Man never is, but always to be blessed.

NOVEMBER 10, 2012

From a daughter who has a mother with Alzheimer's

Last night when I saw my mom I noticed her hair was flat on her head. Lately I have noticed this happening more often. Every day it is a new experience. I honestly never know what to expect, but I am learning. I think of it this way, what would Mom want? So I have made a mental list. She would want her nails painted. Check. She would want purple clothes to wear. Check. She would want cute shoes. Check. She would want magazines to read. Check. She would want it to be clean where she lives. Check. She would also want makeup and her hair fixed. So, I fix her hair. I never did her hair in the past, but I am learning to be a pretty good hair stylist. I notice as I brush her hair that it is getting thinner and thinner. It is just like her, it is slowly fading away. Another silly reminder, although so insignificant. But, still an analogy all the same. So, I try and fix it and cover all the thin spots. I keep trying to fix her too. I just can't seem to let her go, not yet anyway. Thank you, God that she still knows who I am.

I brushed my mother's hair.

I brushed and curled her hair

Now the color of a cultured pearl

She sat so still as if a small girl waiting for dance recital

Every now and then she would say to me

I have to get ready

I have friends to see

I took each curl and sprayed it lightly,

twisted it around my finger

I did it over and over

I wanted the time with her to linger

When it was all done

She looked into her mirror

She reached into her makeup bag

Put on her favorite lipstick

Licked her lips

Looked at me

And said...

Come give me a kiss.

Don't I look pretty?

NOVEMBER 12, 2012
Thank you for the Army, Navy, Air Force, Marines, All Veterans

When visiting my mom today, I walked in and saw all the AD patients sitting in the living area, listening to a gentleman playing his accordion. It was a golden color and a little tarnished. You could tell he had given many hours of joy to people while playing this beautiful piece of music machinery. He played all their old favorites, "Take me out to the ballgame," "I'll be seeing you," "You are my sunshine," and many more. There were only two gentlemen in the whole group and the rest were ladies. Some of the ladies had instruments such as tambourines and other smaller, easier noisemakers. They all seemed to be very excited and joyful. The accordion player would walk around and sing to each person at different times. I heard some beautiful voices when I was in that room. I could only imagine how some had probably sung in their church choir at one time. Another moved her body while in her wheel chair, and she raised her arms to the beat of the music. I saw her in my mind's eye as a young girl dancing around the ballroom with her date. All of these seniors at one time had their own story of life and love, and it showed in the movements of their body to the music as it was played. The gentleman who sat and only listened, and smiled occasionally, did not move or say much, he just sat there. The accordion player asked if there were any Veterans there. At that moment the quiet man smiled and whispered, lightly raising his hand. Just a little. The accordion player walked over to hear him better. He asked what branch he served in. The man took his time, as if to remember, and then it was like his memory clicked in, a smile crossed his face and he sat up straighter in his chair. He could only get his voice a little above a whisper but proudly said, "The Navy." The accordion player immediately took his instrument in his hands, and played the most beautiful rendition of "Eternal Father (Strong to Serve). As soon as he was finished playing, he walked up to the man in his wheelchair and saluted him. He then thanked him for his service to our country. The proud Veteran smiled and sat even straighter.

I have never felt so proud for my country, so proud for a Veteran. He still, even with the disease of Alzheimer's, remembered what branch of service he had served in, for the United States of America.

Thank you to all the Veterans today and let us NEVER FORGET the price paid for our freedom and those who served!

NOVEMBER 18, 2012

Sometimes in your life you are forced to deal with abusive and obtrusive people. It is not something one would choose to do but sometimes it is unavoidable due to certain circumstances. My daughter, Mindy Michelle Stevens, never ceases to amaze me with her steadfast calmness in the realm of irrationality by some individuals. My mother was also blessed to have some awesome and very faithful individuals as neighbors. You can truly see God working in them. Normally, a day like today would have me very upset, but I am very thankful that this ends one more chapter in our life and in my mom's life. It clearly shows, again, that she is safe, she is loved and that God is controlling all of the things going on in my family's lives. I feel a true peace I have not felt in a long time, and I am not under the influence of one drop of wine. xoxoox

NOVEMBER 23, 2012
Thanksgiving with Mom, Mindy, and Jane.

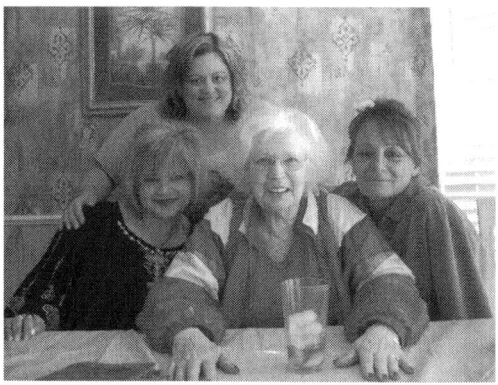

NOVEMBER 25, 2012
From a daughter who has a mother with AD
When I first entered the facility where my mom is staying. I noticed everyone had a shadow box by his or her door. Mindy and I filled Moms up with articles from the DPD. We also placed pictures of her and Murray inside of it, her letters of commendations, etc., a few of her favorite dried flowers and her name plate that came from her desk. I noticed and reviewed everyone's shadow box. Each one of the people, who now were a mere shadow of themselves, had once been like you and me. They were vibrant, healthy people who had a special place in a family, a career, and were loved. I noticed in Larry's shadow box was a picture of a robust handsome man, tall, broad shoulders, with a big cowboy hat on. It looked as though he lived on a ranch at one time. Many times when I would visit, Larry would smile when I walked in and wave his hand to say "Hello." He rarely spoke. All the women sat around Larry, he loved the attention. I noticed the last few times I was there, he was lying in bed. Last night I asked the head nurse where he was. I was told that Larry had passed away. I did not even know his last name. I had only been around this man a few times, yet his passing

affected me deeply. I found myself asking how long he had been there. Questions and fears grasping at my heart. It takes such little effort to love people and to get close to them, especially when they are so fragile. These are the times when I ask myself, "How can anyone take advantage of those who cannot take care of themselves?" The elderly, children, animals; are all beings who depend on others for their survival. It is so easy to love them. I barely knew this man, yet his passing causes me sorrow for what he had and then lost to Alzheimer's.

When I get sad about Larry being gone I will just imagine he is on his horse, cowboy hat on and riding towards the loving arms of God. Ride on Larry! xoxo

NOVEMBER 29, 2012

Thanks Hope Stewart, you are always answering every concern I have about Mom. God is giving me back some "hope" that I have lost since the ongoing illness of my beloved mother. In the words of a very wise Jewish girl *"In spite of everything I still believe that people are really good at heart. I simply can't build up my hopes on a foundation consisting of confusion, misery and death."* -Anne Frank, *The Diary of a Young Girl*

NOVEMBER 30, 2012
The lighter side of AD

When visiting my mom last night, she lit up like a Christmas tree when first seeing me walk in the door. She was lying in bed. As she turned over to see me, she looked so beautiful. Her skin was silky smooth, her hair was white like newly fallen snow, and it glistened. Her eyes were so bright they almost lit up her face. She was exceptionally beautiful. She started running her fingers through my hair telling me how pretty she thought I was. She kept saying how thick my hair was, how pretty it looked. Did I get it cut? I was her pretty little girl. As usual I was biting back the tears. I knew she was seeing me as a child. I guess God decided to jump in and help me out so I would not fall apart and start bawling like a baby. Her next question was, "Where are all my other children?" Since I am an only child, I said, "Mom, I ran them all off so I would be your only child!" We laughed and laughed and then she whacked me across the arm.
In life, laughter truly is the 'best medicine.'

DECEMBER 5, 2012
My mother/my Hero and her Alzheimer's

I found myself looking through her files at home. I was searching for things for her party on Saturday. Our Mothers, I believe, are whom we envision we will most likely be like. My mother was always the most beautiful creature on earth to me. I had to have been adopted. I was chubby, round faced and quite awkward. On the other hand my mother was slim, beautiful and quite graceful. Funny thing is, she thought she was awkward and anything but graceful. I did not know this until just recently from reading all of her entries of her writings found around the house. She was anything but what she thought. I found she almost had a 4.0 grade point average from El Centro College. I found her Police Academy graduation papers. I found stacks of commendations, I found letters from large companies, one of those from American Express thanking her for saving their company huge amounts of money. In 1972 Police Chief Dyson speaks about how there are now seven policewomen on the force for Dallas, June Mcline and Rosemary Birdwell, were one of the first to be assigned to criminal investigations. Women were now eligible to compete for all ranks within the department.

Dallas Policewomen played a vital role and my mother was one of them. This country girl who spent her childhood years growing up on a farm in Arkansas picking cotton, growing her own food for the dinner meals, and milking a cow. She now had a grown daughter lying on a closet floor in awe, looking through all these papers of Mom's prior accomplishments long after the farming days had gone by.

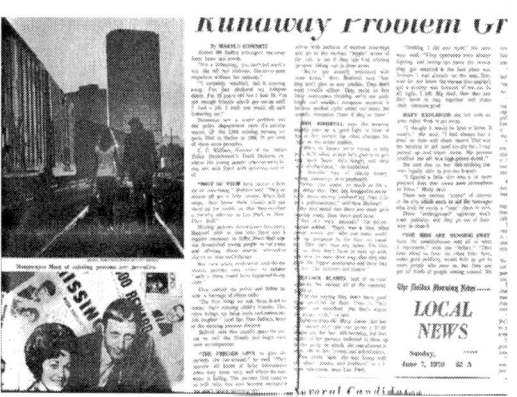

I wish she had shared with me all these accomplishments when I could have looked her in the eye and told her how proud I was of her. How she was a pioneer, how she was my HERO. I don't think I ever saw one of these articles. My mother was very content just being a mother and felt blessed having a good job with good pay. She was not out to win any awards. This was the type of person she was.

On Saturday I will have all of her paper clippings, commendations, write ups, pictures, everything I could find. I hope down deep inside she will know what she means to me. "The gender is different, but the dedication is the same"

DECEMBER 6, 2012

Mom's surprise birthday party! I am getting more excited every day. If I have not called you back or sent you directions, PLEASE contact me. I have so much in my head right now; I have no space to remember to eat my dark chocolate. That should explain exactly how busy this little, tiny mind of mine is. I think someone should feel really sorry for me, come over and force-feed me some chocolate before I go into shock. P.S. I am not kidding! Well half way, maybe.

DECEMBER 8, 2012

I want to take this time to thank everyone who came to Mom's party. I wish I could do it by name but I think Facebook would think I was spamming on here. I asked every-one to go around the room and tell some incident they could remembered that involved Mom. It was fun, sentimental and at times hilarious. Sometimes it was very emotional. My mom did not have Alzheimer's today. She knew everyone, she was sharp, she was funny, and she was enchanting. If I had dreamed of a way I would have wanted her to be, it would have been the way she was today. God gave her this day, God gave her friends this day to remember her by, and God gave the family this day. I will never be more thankful than I was today. I saw the genuine love, friendship, and camaraderie of co-workers, neighbors, friends, and family. If I was ever blessed, this will go down as one of those days. xoxoox

The most awesome caregivers and owners of the best caregiving company in the world are Patsy Corliss and her sister Barbara McVicker. Clear Choice Senior Care was the impetus for helping Mindy and I save my mother. Thank you. xoox

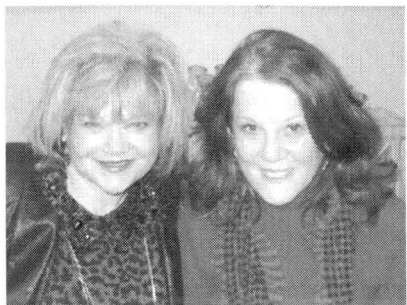

DECEMBER 9, 2012

The birthday party looked like a retired Dallas Police Officers reunion get together! Wow, wow, wow! 30 or so of some of the most awesome, loving and kind people in the world. Many thanks to so many people.

DECEMBER 19, 2012 AT 11:48PM

The daughter of a mother who has Alzheimer's (I don't remember having a birth-day party)

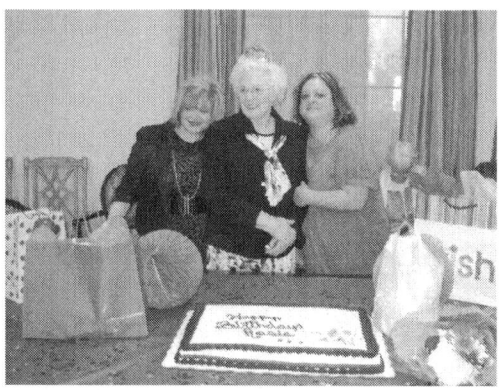

Mindy and I saw Mom today. We took her a Starbucks coffee and some pumpkin bread. As we walked in, I noticed her hair was messy and her clothes a little mis-matched. I know this has more to do with me than with her. She had on her favorite comfortable shoes I bought her a few months ago, and her long white socks to keep her feet warm. When she saw us, she had the same sweet, wide grin and her eyes opened up and welcomed us.

She was just finishing her lunch, but gladly took the pumpkin bread. We mentioned her party from last Saturday and she asked, "Were we going to give her a party?" I knew then she had already forgotten. My heart sank in my chest. Why wasn't I use to this by now? I pulled out my cell phone and showed her pictures of everyone that came that day. She was ecstatic to see all the faces. She pretended she remembered the party but I knew better.

After finishing her bread we walked to her room. I worked a little on her Christmas tree and moved things around. I checked on her clothes, her toiletries and her magazines. I found the bag of birthday cards she had not opened from her party. Mindy and I sat with her while she opened each one. She loved her cards and she remembered most of the people's names, but she did not remember them being there. She knew they were by the pictures and cards. I explained how much she was loved. How far people had traveled to see her.

I began to ask her why she had never told me about her commendations, her letters from parents thanking them for finding a lost child, companies writing about how she saved them from exploitation, why? She answered, "Mary, I was just doing my job." I said, "Mom, you are my hero and I am so proud of you!" She looked at me and tears came to her eyes. She reached out and pulled me to her face and kissed me. She said, "I guess I did do a good job, didn't I?"

My mother was always a very unpresuming woman.

It is no surprise to anyone who reads my blog how much I love and admire my mom. I want to protect her from this disease and yet there is NO protection and I feel helpless at times. Tonight I feel particularly helpless.

This is one of those nights I want to run and hold her and tell her everything will be ok like she used to tell me. But, I know it won't be. I have to accept there will be nights like this for me.

One thing I can be grateful in knowing is, she does not feel this loneliness. The mind of an Alzheimer's patient does not have these feelings and if so it is only for a few minutes.

I can be grateful that she is only lonely for a few fleeting minutes. This gives me some solace when I worry that she may be missing me, the passing time, the seasons, and her memories.

Good night, Mom
See you in my dreams! xoxox

JANUARY 7, 2013
I am on my way to the hospital. Mom has been transported there by ambulance. Please send lots of prayers her way.

JANUARY 8, 2013

It never ceases to amaze me how much my mother is loved. I cannot keep up with the emails, texts, phone calls, etc. from those who are concerned about her. Calls go as far back as friends who have known her for 40 years or more, co-workers, neighbors, and even physicians who adored her. If love could have a name it would be Rosie, I believe. There seems to be no change. More and more tests. All I know is that my mom is not her usual self, even her "usual Alzheimer's self." I continue to ask God for a complete healing. xoxoox

My mother has Alzheimer's.... The even scarier side of Alzheimer's

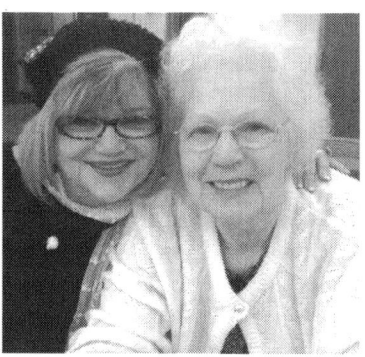

I was sitting there getting my nails done. I had just enough time to get to my counseling session. I had so much I wanted to discuss with him. So many fears concerning Mom. So much joy we had all experienced over the holidays. I could not wait to get feedback about what I was learning about this horrible debilitating disease. Was I a good student? Was I learning how to master the pain it brought me, the sadness, the loneliness? My cell phone rang and I noticed the call coming from the "nurse's station," I started to panic. This was not going to be a social call, not at this hour. I picked it up and I heard the nurse tell me Mom was being transported to the Emergency room. My breath left my body in one swoop. I froze. Then I gathered my thoughts and asked, "Why, what happened?" I don't think I really heard what was said, after, "She had a seizure like episode." When it comes to my loved ones I lose all sense of reality. I am not a good nurse when it comes to the people I love. I become more like the patient in need of a tranquilizer.

I was told I would need to come and bring her insurance cards; they were unable to locate them. I was there in less than ten minutes. As I pulled up I did not even park in a parking place. I just parked. I ran inside past all the special codes that I could not remember and luckily my innate "sane self" took over. Mom was being wheeled out. She looked pale, glassy eyed, weak and old. She had not looked old to me, ever. I asked her if she was cold. She just stared at me. I asked the attendant if she was cold. All I could think of was that my mother was cold and needed to be covered. They assured me she would be warm in the ambulance. I did not cry. I patted her and said I would see her at the hospital. Again, I was told where she would be going and directions. Again, I heard the words being spoken but they did not register. All I could hear was what was in my head. I don't want my mom to be cold and I want her to be OK.

I started calling people I loved. People I knew would be there for me. People I knew loved my mother. This gave me comfort.

Mindy came to the house to pick me up and we drove to the hospital together. There was Mom in a room being attended to. She was not herself. She was not even her "Alzheimer's self." I would have settled for even that at that very moment. I looked at her. For the first time in my life she looked smaller to me, weaker, frailer, a little scared. She was not making jokes, and she was not the tough Rosie.

I am losing her. I finally admitted that fact to myself. Maybe not today, but yes, I am losing her.

The brain is the major organ in the body. It controls all the other organs. I hate this disease. It is robbing me of my mother's smile, her laughter, and her life. One day it will take away her ability to know my name, to swallow and to breathe.

I have to ask myself each day if I am willing to let her go and today the answer is "No." Maybe tomorrow I will be strong enough to say yes, but today, God, can I keep her today?

Please get better Mom. I need you.

JANUARY 9, 2013
I am at the hospital. Mom has 102.7 temperature. Neither the nurses nor I are able to wake her up. The staff is saying she has just checked out for the day. I have tried bribing her with everything to get her to open her eyes. Never in my entire life have I seen my mom this helpless. Prayers appreciated for Mom to wake up! xoxo

JANUARY 10, 2013

Mom's temp is over 103 and she has been diagnosed with pneumonia in her right upper lung. They are not even sure this is where the infection stems from. They are even considering sepsis. (God forbid) She still won't open her eyes and is unresponsive. Before leaving tonight I wanted her to know I was there, and that I was leaving and I loved her. It was hard to find a place on her that was not hooked up to some contraption. I took her hand and rubbed her fingers. I started singing, "You are my sunshine, my only sunshine, you make me happy, when skies are gray." At that time I heard a slight whisper, she was singing the song with me. We finished the song together. She never opened her eyes except for a tiny slit when I said "goodbye" and that I loved her. She then said in a little hoarse whisper, "I love you too" Only a mother can love you like no other. Please don't take my sunshine away. xoxo

JANUARY 10, 2013

Wow, my cup runneth over with love to all those who care so much for my mom and for our family. I will keep everyone posted. If love and prayers could heal, she would be up and running. I can feel the care and compassion in every post. Thank you. xoxoxoox

JANUARY 10, 2013

"All God's angels come to us disguised." - James Russel Lowell
I honestly could not keep up with the calls, emails and texts today concerning Mom. Prayer after prayer. I have witnessed it personally when doing my nursing. In all reality I truly felt Mom would not live through the week. Today she opened her eyes and sat up in her hospital bed. She is still weak, still a little disoriented, but the difference between yesterday and today, to put it bluntly, is a miracle of pure unadulterated love and the power of prayer. Thank you angels. xoooxox Mom and "Dr. Ally" ...commonly

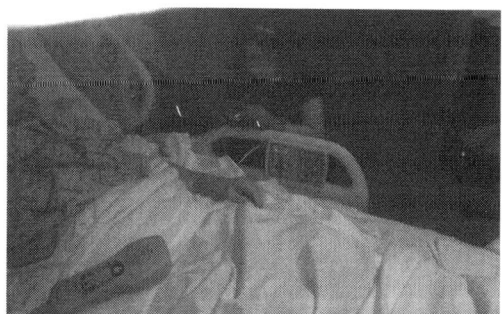

referred to as Kenady. By the way grape jelly makes an awesome medicinal product. Caution=keep lid on.

JANUARY 13, 2013

Mom had a little bit of a setback today. Mindy Michelle Stevens was the champion and stayed with her much of the day. I did the quarterbacking. Our favorite caregiver from Clear Choice Senior Care Angeline, was there today for me, Mom and Mindy. Janice took me out to have some time to feel ok about the world. Thanks Janice Vestal Boudreau. So, with ANGELine, my best friend, and my baby girl in my corner, I was able to laugh for a few hours and just put mom in God's hands. The best place for anyone to be. Get better Mom. I love you!

JANUARY 14, 2013

Alzheimer's patients have what is called a "drop," meaning their symptom progress at a rapid level. Sometimes this will level off in time and they will get to the point where they were before the "drop." Mom has had a definite drop. She no longer has much of a desire to feed herself or to do basic things as she did before. I am not a fool, I know how the disease progresses. I knew there was a chance this may happen. Hopefully she will be released tomorrow and go into skilled nursing. My hope now is for her to go back to her "before" condition. With the disease of Alzheimer's you will settle for crumbs, because even then, they become pieces of gold to be treasured. xoxo

JANUARY 15, 2013

Mom was not released today, she suffered another seizure. I have a peace about this or maybe I am just in denial. Either way, I am no longer afraid of the outcome. I feel totally surrounded by a bubble of love and understanding. I believe everything that happens in this life has a purpose. God will direct me on exactly what I am to learn from all this. One of my favorite writers is Helen Keller. Think of all the obstacles surrounding her and yet she found beauty all around her, and she could not even see.
"Although the world is full of suffering, it is full also of the overcoming of it." -Helen Keller

JANUARY 16, 2013

My mother has Alzheimer's....five steps to the goal line.
I am a strong woman when it comes to people I love. This is when I can be strong, nurturing and level headed. But, aren't we all like that? Let someone get around a mother bear's cubs and see what she does, she will eat your face off and not think a

thing about it. We women have this innate ability to protect those we love and we will do it in a heartbeat. I always knew my mother was strong, resourceful, independent and someone to be admired. I see her now as someone who depends on me to be the strong one for her. When I was with her last night she looked so frail, so elderly, so confused. I saw my own immortality.

Mom has been told to stay in her bed due to the seizures. I left the room to talk to the caregiver. The alarm started going off on her bed. We ran into the room. Mom was trying to get out of bed. Everyone was telling her to get back in bed. Mom said, "I need to go to the bathroom." Everyone was saying, "No, you are too weak." I said, "Let her go if she wants to!" She looked over at me with big eyes and stood taller. It took three people to help her to the restroom. She was hooked up to machines and we were all holding something but she accomplished her mission. Later, when we got her in bed, I looked at her and she seemed different, not as frail, not as weak and not as afraid. Those five tiny steps, mission accomplished! She knew she had done it! She said, "I want to get out of here, I hate this place." I said, "You will leave here tomorrow, I promise!" She smiled.

They are releasing her at 3:30 today by ambulance to rehabilitation.

Don't ever tell someone they can't do something, ever, ever, ever. The spirit is a fragile thing. I was there at that particular time for a reason. I was there to be her voice and to push for her independence. Alzheimer's is teaching me so much about mental illness, so much about life. These people are not deaf or dumb. They can hear what you are saying about them and to them. They may not remember five minutes later, but the spirit remembers.

It is just like with us so called "normal" people. We all need reinforcement, encouragement, and love.

You go Mom. RAH, RAH, RAH!

JANUARY 17, 2013
My mother has Alzheimer's...being grateful for the teenie tiny things... :)
Mom was carried by ambulance to a rehabilitation unit. I kept my promise. YAY! Although she does not remember the promise I made, I do. I walked in this afternoon and she was sitting in a wheelchair. I pretended in my head it was a Queen's throne. I am

an only child. I have a great imagination!

As I walked up to her I noticed she had on some of my readers. I think they are 225 plus. I said, "Mom, where are your glasses?" By the way, these are purple animal print, foo- foo, and rhinestone glasses. They are just for when I am at home and to read small print. I loaned them to her because she lost her glasses at the hospital, her prescription glasses. I was sure she could not see a dang thing in these glasses unless it was as small as an ant. A person she looked at would have resembled a blurry anomaly of a human.

She said she could see fine. I knew better.

She reached into her pocket and told me she won $25.00 at bingo and a coupon. With Alzheimer's you don't know what is real or imagined. I noticed something in her pocket and sure enough she had won a free hair styling at the beauty shop where I have her hair styled twice a month. She was ecstatic, as was I.

I went to the room they have her in until she is better and back on her feet. There were her "old" glasses hanging on the blinds. I knew that was where they would be. I walked back, took off the readers, and put the prescription glasses on her face. She smiled.

The nurse told her it was time for dinner and off she went, and off I went to get her some jammies for the night. When I returned she was in the dining room. I walked up to her and asked her if she enjoyed her meal. She looked at my new scarf and said, "Where did you get that ugly scarf?" I told her I got it for her and we both laughed. Maybe I should not have found her glasses. LOL

She goes from the wheelchair to the cane to walking again. Even if she hates my new scarf, I will still be grateful for the teeniest tiniest things called improvement when it comes to this disease.

Love you Mom and no, you cannot borrow my new scarf.

JANUARY 18, 2013
My mother has Alzheimer's. What a wonderful world it would be...If...

The only way I can describe the disease of Alzheimer's is to ask you to remember what you had for dinner two weeks ago on a certain day at a certain time. Your mind goes completely blank. You try and try to recall, but 90% or more of us cannot remember what we ate for dinner two nights ago. Try living in a world like this on a daily basis. It is a new world every five minutes. The reason Alzheimer's patients remember people, is because as babies we learn "faces," and recognition of people by their faces. This is usually the last thing to go for an Alzheimer's patient. They may lose the ability to talk, eat and even do simple bodily functions, but they will still recognize certain people even if they cannot remember names. My mom gets Mindy and I confused at times and while in the hospital she did not recognize Mindy; an hour later she did. After the age of 80 years old, half of the population has some type of Dementia. Please keep that in mind when Grandma or Grandpa asks you the same question more than once.

The laws need to be changed. At the present time they have not caught up with this horrible disease. This disease is cunning and powerful and can eat your loved one alive, bit by bit. There is no known cure and no way to slow it down. This opens up the door to all kinds of abuse and neglect to the person who is suffering.

As I get older, I realize I am not exempt from death; too bad it took me this long. Our older population, due to the baby boom generation, is growing by leaps and bounds. Every time I forget anything these days I ask myself, will I succumb to Alzheimer's? What a wonderful world it would be if we all truly cared so much for one another that we knew we would be cared for no matter what disease we might succumb to, what ailment we might have, or what may happen to us. I would like to think or I hope that I can be a deposit into the account for my mom and not a withdrawal from her bank of life.

Love you Mom.

JANUARY 21, 2013
As usual Hope Stewart did her famous multi-tasking today and came out like a champ when it came to Mom's needs. Hope, your name suits you so well. It is people like you, Scott and Tiffany that give "hope" to families that are dealing with a loved one who suffers from a debilitating disease. You guys give Mindy and I a chance to take a breath and relax for a minute or two. If I had a bucket of blessings I would pour them all over you. xoxoox

JANUARY 23, 2013
Alzheimer's ...can teach you about love.
Ever had a bad dream and you awake and think, oh, was I dreaming? Yep, I am having a bad dream. Thank God, that was only a dream, a horrible one. Then that feeling of

relief comes over you.

Alzheimer's is that bad dream you never awake from and the whole family has the same dream. I can just imagine how it is for the participant who lives it day in and day out. I hear people say, "Well, she does not know, so that is a blessing." I guess if AD has any blessings we would have to count that as half of one.

Life is not supposed to be easy. What would we learn if it was? I think I have always been one of those people who finds my glass half full instead of half empty. I try to imagine my mother without Alzheimer's, but then would someone else have to suffer with it if she did not? I learned a long time ago that nothing, absolutely nothing, happens by chance. God has his hand in everything. I am actually supposed to be grateful. Who came up with that concept.

If I look back at the big picture I can see there are many blessings that have come from her disease. It is against my analytical mind to do this but it coincides with my spiritual side. I could have lost her in 2010 when she got lost for 16 hours, and was found by a police officer in Argyle, Texas. Remember, nothing, absolutely nothing, happens by chance in God's world.

This has given us over two more years plus with her. I prayed that night that she would be found; I did not care how sick she was or how sick she would get. God answered my prayer.

I continue to try and count the blessings. Some days when she refuses to take her meds, can't walk or she looks at me and acts as though she has a hard time remembering who I am, those are the hard times. My self-pity, my anger, my fear, and my loneliness tries to eat up any joy for the day.

Then there are the days like today, when people who genuinely cared about the health and outcome of my mom surrounded Mindy and me. They are lovingly there for me when I have to consider tough decisions. Any terminal illness has its devastation and sadness. If we take time to look around us and see the love from a friend, a caregiver, a Pastor, a nurse, even a family member of another Alzheimer's patient, we can see the true light of love.

Love that only asks to be given away, just take it. The only cost is my acceptance of it by another human being.

I accept love in all forms today, for Mom and for me. I am seeing the light of love in the darkness of Alzheimer's. Quite frankly, it is Heavenly.

JANUARY 24, 2013
Today (so far) LOL
Mom would not take her meds got a call, got me out of bed
I am not above bribery
Or begging if need be
Red fingernail polish and painting nails work just fine too, you see
The dog ate a whole pack of double bubble even got it in her hair
Telling Kenady about the gum I don't dare. (It was hers)
The teenage girl next door came over when I pulled up
She needed some understanding and some love
My days are never boring, or without someone in need
I always seem to be the one to fill the space if someone feels empty
I consider this a blessing a gift one might say but in doing this I get much more than
I EVER GIVE AWAY.
1/24/13

JANUARY 28, 2013
I want to go and spend some time with my dad. I have been so stressed lately due to moms Alzheimer's. But then guilt settles in about leaving my mom for a few days. When you hear the word "stressed" from so many people that love you, I guess it is time to listen. My favorite love, swimming, has taken a back seat to Mom's affairs. In my quest to "fix" everything, I am losing myself. It is very hard for me to ask for help or to admit I am not on top of things. This has been a 28-month, ongoing, everyday type of thing. Writing has been one way of being able to let out some of the pain and loss I feel inside. The rest I internalize. I have read how caregivers can sometimes get as sick as, or sicker than the person requiring care. I don't want to be this way. My question is, how can a daughter NOT be intertwined into her mother's life? How can a daughter disconnect from her mother's needs? I wake up thinking about her and I go to bed thinking about her. I feel so extremely sorry for her and her condition. If anyone has any words of experience please share these with me. No, I am not perfect, I am far from it, imagine that!

FEBRUARY 5, 2013
Just moved mom from her old room to a new room closer to the nurse's station with

an awesome view of the patio, and dining area. I was told it could not be done. Please don't tell an adult you can't do something for his or her momma. Then we will just have to show you! Mom loves her new room. (Smooches Mommy)

FEBRUARY 7, 2013
Mom's new room in the world of Alzheimer's... :)

My mom is like a social butterfly, she flies here, and she flies there. The little pollinator, I call her. To some of the other occupants she is their nurse, others, their best friend and to others she is the police officer on call. I have seen a new side to her, a more nurturing side. I have seen her try to cover wounds with Band-Aids, push occupants in wheel chairs, and give advice. In other words, she keeps herself quite busy. After the recent dip in her condition I was worrying she would not recover to her "normal" self. At least what we in the family consider "normal".

When moving her items to the new room I noticed other occupants coming in and out of her room. Each one would wheel themselves by and introduce themselves to me. "Hi, I am so and so, glad to have you here," and then wheel away. This went on for quite some time. It was like neighbors introducing themselves to the new neighbor in the neighborhood. So thoughtful, so caring and so kind. The only difference is, I had met them many times before. I pretended I had not. It was fun in a way. I always find joy in these wonderful people.

To them, Mom was a new resident in a new room. I felt such a warmness come over me. I have lived on my block for over ten years and know two of my neighbors. Mom had been in her room less than thirty minutes and all of her old neighbors introduced themselves as new neighbors in less than fifteen minutes. They were genuinely concerned about their "NEW" tenant.

Mom invited each one in, showed them her furniture, her surroundings and they made jokes like a bunch of teenagers would. It was quite charming to say the least. It was dinnertime now and I could hear all the occupants sitting around the tables discussing the meal for the day. I turned my head to the other side and looked out her window to see the trees and the benches. Yes, Mom was where she needed to be, safe and sound and she was the newest kid on the block. Just for that little bit of time, Alzheimer's time.

Be safe little butterfly. xoxoox

FEBRUARY 17, 2013

This is me and Mom after a meal together. She is still so beautiful. In this picture she is all natural, no makeup. I heart emoticon her! Time with her is so precious.

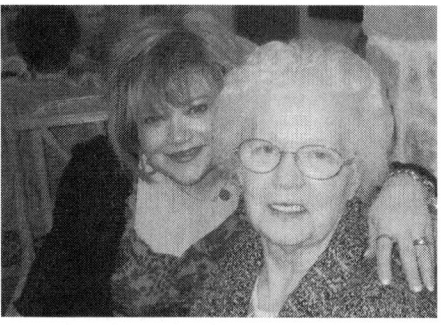

"Whatever you do, do it all for the glory of God".
1 Corinthians 10:3

FEBRUARY 17, 2013

My mom has Alzheimer's, I wish I had a magic key.

I visited Mom last night. She was sitting at the desk looking at a valentine's card. She read this card over and over and over again. The girls at the center were talking to us, and to me, as she kept reading this card over and over again. I asked her if she had read my card, she gave me a glance and look bewildered. I repeated I had brought her a card and sugar free candy on Valentine's Day. She just looked at me. I went to get her card. It was about 16 inches tall and very colorful. I had to get her attention twice to show it to her. I asked her if she wanted any of the candy. She said, "Yes." I asked her if she wanted her nails painted but we could not find the polish so I asked if I could fix her hair, she said "Yes." I pulled out all the things I needed and they let me fix her hair at the front desk so she could still be engaged with everyone. She never spoke unless I spoke to her first and then it was one-word answers. I took each piece of her hair and twirled it around the comb, remembering all the times she had curled my hair as a chlld. I loved touching her soft shiny silver hair and watching it curl and then glisten in the light. She barely spoke four words. She was still reading the same card. The same one she was reading when I came in. Maybe twenty words on one side of the card with a valentine print on the front. What was she seeing? What was she thinking? I often wonder what her Alzheimer's mind actually sees that our minds don't. When I finished with her hair I put a little makeup on her and everyone told her how beautiful she looked. Someone asked her whom she was getting all fixed up for. She always looks to me for her answers. I asked, "Is it Murray Katzen?" She did not say anything. I could tell she did not process whom I was speaking of. I asked if it was Ray Birdwell and she smiled and said, "Yes." Since this is my dad, I knew her disease was progressing. It has been over 40 years since she has seen my dad. I walked her to her room and helped her get her pajamas on. I have to instruct her what to do. It is almost robotic, but she is able to perform the function. She has to have the guidance or she is lost.

I asked her to lie in the bed and I would tuck her in. She would be my little baby and I would be the Mommy tonight. She liked that. I put pink fluffy soft booties on her feet and covered her with two huge comforters. I got in bed beside her and told her she was the best mom anyone could have and then I kissed her. I said, "I love you Mom" and she said, "I love you Mary." As usual, I was fighting back my tears.

I wish I had a magic key to unlock her brain for just one hour. If God could give me 60 minutes to ask her what she needs from me to make her more comfortable, make this more bearable, what a miracle that would be.

At this point I can only guess what she needs from me.

"Now faith is the substance of things hoped for, the evidence of things unseen."
Unknown

FEBRUARY 28, 2013
My mother has Alzheimer's...what a "good" day is like; cherish those.
Mindy and I went to see Mom today. When we walked in Mom was wearing all purple, her favorite color. She even had on my purple readers. A reminder that next week we would go and get her some new glasses. Her hair was fixed with her new, shorter length, and when she saw us she smiled from one ear to the other. She was sitting next to a (at one time) prominent attorney who now suffers with the same disease she does. So many of the residents she shares space with were once such vital members of society, each contributing to this world. Each one had a family, at one time, having hopes and dreams just like all of us. I sometimes wish I could have one day with each one of them in the "before" Alzheimer's life. One of the many things I have learned through my mother's illness is that sick, well, young or old we all deserve dignity and respect. The residents in her ward gathered in the activity room and each had a songbook and tambourines, and we all began to sing some old time favorites. Mindy got up from her chair and began to dance with Mom as she sat there. Mindy twirled around the chair and pretended to dance with Mom. My mom laughed and I laughed, and others

giggled too. It was a priceless moment. It was one that will be in my memory forever; cherished.

Of course my Mom always notices my jewelry. She noticed my newest flower ring I got from Marilou. She said, "I want that and I want your purse too." Then Mindy said, "I want a ring like that too." I said, "I will get you both a ring but no one gets my purse." I explained I would have no way to carry my things home. My mom promptly said, "Put your stuff in a bag!" We all laughed again.

Yes, today was a good day. It was filled with laughter and I watched my daughter and my mother dance together for the very first time. :)

Thank you God for today and for my beautiful and gracious mother, and my sweet and loving, playful daughter.

"God causes everything to work together for the good of those who love God".
Romans 8:28 NLT

MARCH 11, 2013
I am her daughter, the abyss of Alzheimer's.
Janice, my BFF and I had a great time at North Park Mall yesterday shopping. She always grounds me, lifts me up, and helps me to remember I am a beautiful woman. I still have wants, desires, and there is life beyond my mother's disease. Janice helped her own mother who had a debilitating disease until the day she succumbed to it. She has been where I am. She too is the daughter of a mother who got lost in the unknown disease realm of life. This makes us kindred spirits.

I went to see Mom after I left North Park. I had a sugar-free chocolate candy for her, her favorite. When I walked in they were in the dining room. I walked up behind her and hugged her. She barely gave me any recognition. I noticed she had on a tiara. I remarked about her tiara and she acknowledged that yes, she was wearing one. She only looked at me once. Her hands were shaking a little and she had dropped some food on herself. I asked if she had a napkin and could I get her one. She immediately reached for her neighbor's napkin. I wanted to say, "Mom, are you angry at me?" But, I knew this was an ignorant question to ask. I had no idea where she was at that moment, how could I question her motives in seeming cold to me?

I began to show her all the goodies I brought for her. She slowly put each one in her pocket. I wanted to tell her how much I missed her, loved her, and needed her back in my life. I wanted to shake her and say "Wake up! I need you!" I could imagine her waking up like a princess newly kissed by a prince. We would walk out of this place as if she had never had this disease. We would go to lunch and then we would go buy her some new shoes. She would tell me about a bad dream she had and how glad she was to be back home. Then all would be well and we would live happily ever after.

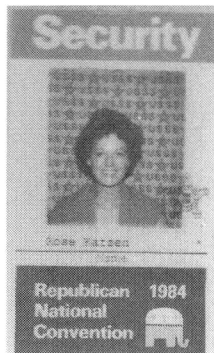

Of course these are only the dreams of a daughter who desperately wants her Momma to be well again, and not lost in some deep immeasurable void never to return.

I came home last night and looked at some of her pictures. I remembered how beautiful she was and still is, how proud I always was of her. Wherever that Alzheimer's mind is, I hope she has no fear and no regrets. I hope above all other things she can still feel my love when I visit her. Even if I cannot "feel" her at times, I want her to still feel my adoring admiration for her sacrifice, courage and strength she exuded every day of her life.

Mom, I am so proud to be your daughter. I will keep reaching for you through the vast chasm of the abyss of Alzheimer's. I will never let go of you.

MARCH 13, 2013

Today I am with family and going to see even more. I feel an uplifting of my spirit, being with those that are closest to my heart and soul. The last time I saw my mom she asked, "When is the last time you saw your dad?" I answered that it had been awhile. She said, "You need to see him." Sometimes even in her disease she is brighter than the brightest star. xoxo

MARCH 18, 2013

Music restores and purifies the spirit...of those suffering.

I was just reading an article about how music is healing to Alzheimer's patients, and those with depression and other ailments. U.S. Rep. Gabrielle Giffords who suffered brain damage after being shot in January of 2011, could not put a three-word sentence together but she could sing several words together in a phrase. They are just now tapping into the healing power of music.

I remember as a young girl how my dad could hear any song on the radio and he would immediately know the name of the song and of the person singing it. We always made a game out of it. I also remember putting his records on the "record player" and playing songs. I suppose that is why I love show tunes. They remind me of a special time my father and I shared together.

I am always trying to find ways to communicate with my mother, as it becomes harder and harder to connect with her. This article gave me some renewed hope. I believe music has a way of transcending the limits and perimeters of Alzheimer's. I remember the times I have heard a song and it reminded me of a love song I heard many years ago. A special song between someone I deeply loved and myself. The songs I heard as a teenager remind me of a particular place and time. We may even remember the exact place we were when we heard it the first time. I can still remember how it felt to play a clarinet. I remember certain moves to certain music. Yes, music is a bond that cannot be broken. We play it at weddings, parties, church, live concerts, while alone in our cars and last but not least, at funerals. We praise God through music. Worship through music is probably when I feel closest to Him.

When my mother was in the hospital a few months ago I shared how we did not think we would be bringing her home, we were able to connect through the beautiful realm of music when I sang "You are My Sunshine" to her. She was so ill with pneumonia and had such a high fever. There were 24 hours we could not wake her. Mindy and I were so tired and finally leaving to get some rest. I walked to Mom's bed. I took her hand and started singing to her. I sang, "You are my sunshine, my only sunshine - you make me happy when skies are gray." She started moving her head very slowly to the music and began to mouth the words without speaking. We had connected through the beautiful realm of music.

I knew this was God's way of saying that she would wake up, and she did the very next morning.

Many times when I go and see my mom they play music for the Alzheimer's patients. They have them touch instruments. I watch their faces as they sing old songs that spark their memories. Sometimes I start dancing. In the beginning I felt silly, now I feel happy and I think it makes the other people there feel happy too. Of course Alzheimer's robs and takes what it wants, but we can choose to take something also. I will take love from it in any way I can.

You are my sunshine, my only sunshine. I have many "sunshine's" in my life today. In the darkness of the tunnel of Alzheimer's I always look for the light at the end. Usually that is where the angels are singing and praising God.

"Make a joyful noise to the Lord, all the earth! Serve the Lord with gladness! Come into his presence with singing"!
Psalm 100:1-2

MARCH 24, 2013
My mother has Alzheimer's ...living with regrets.
During this time of being sick and stuck at home I have had a lot of time on my hands. Having a touch of ADD does not give me the opportunity to just take time to "smell the roses." Well, the last few days I have been forced to keep my butt in bed and be still and quiet.

Last night I started going through piles of pictures and other items for Mom. I came across a picture of her dancing at the birthday of one of the two major loves in her life, Murray Katzen, the other my dad. I think with my mom and dad it was a first love that got lost in bad choices made by both of them, and yet to this day my dad still adores my mother. Who doesn't?

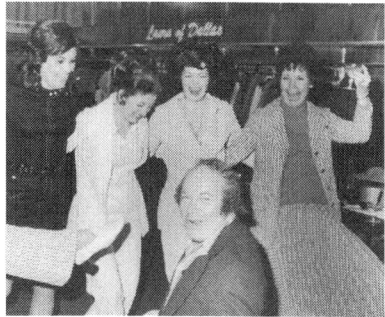

Murray Katzen in front and Mom directly behind him laughing and dancing.

Sometimes I regret not spending more time with my mom. Time I chose in my 30's to spend with my friends. I remember her making references to this often. I thought she was nagging. Why do we have to age to mature?

Mom is in her own little world now, one I cannot explain or define. When I can't visit her, like today, I feel such a gnawing of self-regret. I regret things I cannot take back or change and time I will never get with her again. The B.A., Before Alzheimer's.

Sometimes I feel like the most inept daughter in the world. I have these twirling thoughts in my mind. I could be doing this, I could be doing that. I could join this organization, I could write this Congressman. I could, I do, and I need to do more. Where does it end? When does a daughter feel she has done all she can for her mother who suffers with AD?

And then this idea came to me. Don't campaign against the disease just for today; don't live in any regrets just for today. Instead, I will copy the picture I found of her dancing and laughing (the way she really was) and I will make it as large as I possibly can and take it to her next week.

I will tell her, again, how beautiful she is, how much I love her, and what a champion she is and was for women in the work place. I will tell her this every day for the rest of my life.

Mommies make the best dancers; every daughter believes this to be true.

MARCH 25, 2013
Mindy tucking her Nana into bed Sunday night. Mom will always adore Mindy. I think that is one memory that will never fade. xoxoox

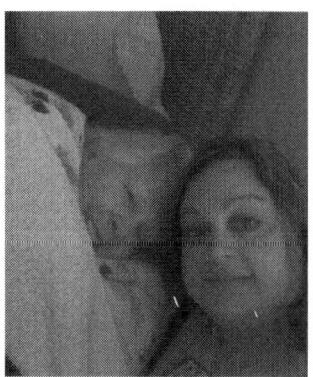

MARCH 28, 2013
Mom, this one today is just for you. I know I will feel your strength, your tenacity, and your courage to overcome any and all obstacles. I have no doubt that every part of you that is in me will be present as I do what needs to be done today. Thank you for being

the strong woman that you were and still are. It helped me to become "her" too! Your loving daughter, Mary. xoxo

MARCH 29, 2013

My Mom has Alzheimer's...She was always there for me at Easter. :)

When I think of Easter, I automatically think of my mom and of the different sounds I would hear in the days before Easter.

My mom was an awesome seamstress as I stated before. She loved that old Singer sewing machine. When the belt would break, she took elastic and made her own "handmade" sewing machine belt. The machine had a beautiful stitch. I can still hear that machine humming if I listen closely. At times that pedal and her foot would move so fast I could not even see her foot moving.

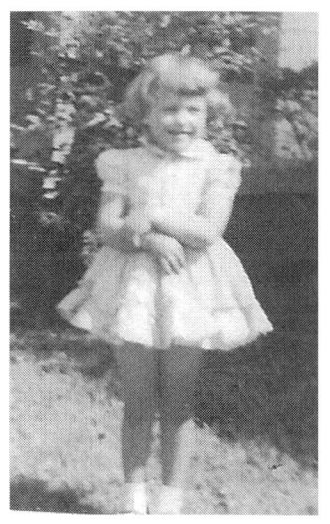

I think she took special effort at Easter to buy me the scratchiest material for my Easter dresses. When I would sit, my dress would spring up like a hooped cup cake. The underwear had to match my dress. Everyone noticed me, but was it the dress or the noise I made?

I had new socks and newly shined shoes and of course a handmade hat, which I removed. Everything on me was handmade except my shoes and socks. I wore gloves that were saved from the year before. I was always a chubby kid in those days, so I most likely did favor a big round Hostess cupcake in either pink or blue.

My mom was always such a frugal person. Growing up in Arkansas as a farm girl and living during the depression changes you. Even after she became a policewoman and made good money, she was still very prudent with her earnings.

She taught me many things about Easter. Of course she taught me about the sacrifice Jesus made, which was first and foremost. She taught me about the love a mother has for her daughter. The love that sacrifices. It sacrifices time, money, energy and finding ways to make your own sewing machine belt so your machine will function. I remember my dad looking at that belt and asking her how did she ever come up with that idea to fix it using that elastic? Her answer was short and sweet.

"Mary had to have her Easter dress."

There are so many things I remember each holiday about my mom. It is like a flood of memories have returned to me. I cannot tell her now because she will not "connect with" what I am talking about. So, I write them down. I know that one day she will know. This is why I write them today.

Thank you for all those homemade dresses Mom. Thank you for telling me all about Jesus and all about Easter too. I was, and still am, blessed to have two wonderful parents.

Happy Easter to Mom and Dad and to anyone reading this. xoxo

MARCH 30, 2013

God answered some awesome prayers for Mindy and I yesterday and I feel a new spirit in my soul. I feel hope, and I feel that God is truly in control of our situation. I almost feel giddy, more than usual. God has placed some very knowledgeable and smart people in our lives. There were times I wanted to give up, literally. Professionals, friends, family and even new friends of less than a year have come to my rescue to help calm my fears and my anger. When you are dealing with losing a loved one, whether to imminent death or to a crippling disease, God can place a cushion of love in that "empty" spot. That hollowed feeling has been filled with so many of you reading this today. Thank you for your love and for always being there for me. xoxox
"He does great things too marvelous to understand. He performs countless miracles."
JOB 5:9 NLT

APRIL 3, 2013
My mom has Alzheimer's...sometimes you find more pieces of the puzzle.
I kept finding pictures of this one particular lady in a lot of Mom's photos. I knew who she was but I could not place her name. So many of Mom's things have been misplaced, her phone turned off and other things that should not have happened. But, this is another story. Then it hit me, this woman was Patsy. She had been at Mindy's wedding, now I knew who she was. If only I could find her number. I went through Mom's address book, which was like going through a puzzle. There were numbers misplaced, in different rows, jumbled and literally written by a mind of an Alzheimer's

sufferer. I found the name Patsy and I called. No one answered, so I left a message. I called back later. We connected. It had been 18 years since we had spoken and briefly seen one another five years ago. She knew only a little of Mom's condition. But, we connected immediately. She had been in Forgery and Theft with Mom for years at the DPD. She gave Mom her retirement party. We knew so many of the same people and police officers. She could tell me things about Mom. It was like I had a little part of my mom with me sitting next to me in the car. I cried when I told her about Mom being lost and found on railroad tracks. We mainly talked about the "good old days, "these are the things I like the best. Again, I learned more about Mom. How can a daughter know so little about her mother? I was telling someone the other day that my mother never patted herself on the back. She just said, "I am nothing special, I am just doing my job." She was very special.

Thank you Lord, for letting me find Patsy. Each time I find another piece of the puzzle I can see who my mother really was. She was a truly an unassuming person. I think the lesson I am supposed to learn, or maybe one of them, is that we each leave a part of ourselves with whomever we meet and have a relationship with. My mother left a piece of herself with everyone she met. I would have never known had it not been for all these pieces that have been put before me. Am I to put together all these pieces until they fit? Will I ever understand the logic behind the disease? I think I am learning as much about myself as I am about my mom through her disease of Alzheimer's. I am just as afraid as she is.

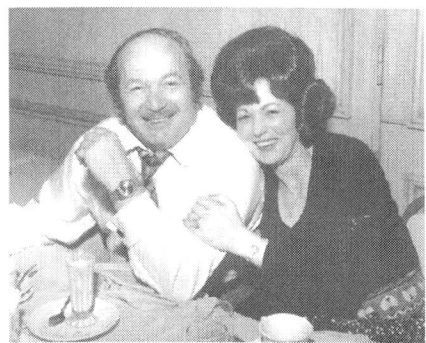

To my mother: Mom, I found a picture of you today with Murray. I wanted to take the picture out of the frame and set you free. But, I knew you were so happy sitting there with him.

Mom, I miss you. xoxox

APRIL 4, 2013

You know when you see that light at the end of the tunnel? Well, it is getting brighter and brighter. I believe that light to be the spirit of God letting me know that all things good are around the corner. I can feel joy returning to my spirit. I believe I have fought the "good" fight for my mother. I also believe that what does not cripple, maim, or eat you alive, makes you stronger. I have always felt myself to be a girl, this last year I think I grew inside to become a woman. A woman to be bargained with. OK, so I am a slow learner. Thanks God for helping me grow! xoxoxo

APRIL 8, 2013

I now have my own web domain for my future book, writings, poems and etc. My very talented daughter, Mindy Michelle Stevens is working on this for me. Then off to an editor and then publisher. My Dad does not know this but since he is an awesome artist, I am going to ask him to do some artwork for me, maybe even get my talented cousin, Barbara Patterson, involved in one of my children's books, "Teacups and Radishes." This idea has been sitting around forever just needing an illustrator. My mother's story is not the only thing I have ever written. It is, however, the impetus to put me into motion to do something with my talents and finally make my dream of publishing a book come true. I give this credit to my mom who has spoken volumes to me through her disease. Thanks Mommy. xoxo

APRIL 10, 2013

Unfortunately, I won't be publicly posting as much. My past poems and posts will be deleted about the journey with my mom and her disease of Alzheimer's. I am getting the manuscript ready for a future book. If I post the past blog, I can't publish a book about it. I definitely want to share my mother with you, the disease of AD, our struggles, and our love through this difficult time. There is life after the diagnosis. If it had not been for so many of you giving me the idea for a book I would have never followed through. If I do get it published, knowing me, I will probably buy all the copies. Just wait a little bit and I will give you your own signed copy. Keep your fingers and eyes crossed for me to find a publisher. xoxoox

APRIL 11, 2013

In the realm of creativity, legalities, feeling loved, and feeling empowered, if things get any better I may bust a gusset. I seem to be surrounded by the most professional people who inspire me to be the best I can be in all areas of my life. To my cousin, Barbara Patterson. I think you saved me from the insane asylum a couple of times these last few years. Although, if they had served chocolate and wine, it might have been a blessing. Now, TGTIF (Thank God tomorrow is Friday)

P.S. What exactly "is" a gusset?

APRIL 12, 2013

I'm not too old to learn new tricks. I can't stop writing what can I say

Today's visit was one of those where the disease of Alzheimer's stretched its ugly nasty head out and said, "Yep, I'm in charge today!" Those are the days I don't visit for very long. It is just the disease and I. It is not my friend, needless to say. So, I kissed her over and over and left. On the way home I stopped at Lowes. Mom loves flowers. I decided that every time I visit her and she is 'absent' I would buy a perennial. Perennial flowers live on year after year. This symbolizes to me that life goes on. No matter where my mother is in her disease, she is still my mother. Alzheimer's cannot steal memories or love. They can return anytime I want them to. I close my eyes and she is there, smiling, dancing, making dinner or curling my hair. Take that Alzheimer's! Now, I will go and plant the first perennial dedicated to my mom who will live forever in my heart.

APRIL 13, 2013

In loving arms

The loving arms of a Nana
Are always open and waiting
Held out for a child's embrace
Always loving and anticipating
Sometimes carrying a warm blanket
Or a cookie sheet right out of the oven
They can be many places.
My favorite memories are those of my two favorite girls
Kissing, laughing, cuddling.
Their own secret society. "shhhh"
Those days, I did not understand it then
But now...being in the "secret" society.
Of all Nana's, GG's or grandmothers
I get it!
In our loving arms,
We are only loving our own little babies all over again. xoxoxo

Mindy at two, with mom encased around her cutting her cake.

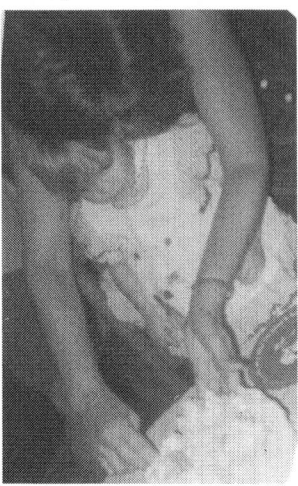

APRIL 22, 2013
Coming home to Momma

Mom and Murray always had Purple Martin houses as long as I can remember. They would forgo having trees in their yard just to welcome these birds every spring. I noticed as moms disease progressed her houses were not being maintained as they should have been. Eventually, they were simply uninhabitable. She got so much pleasure from watching the birds soar, have babies and sing their melodies. They were her babies each spring, hers and Murray's. When Murray passed away in 2000, she still waited each year for them. Purple Martins mate for life and once here, they have their young and then fly back to Brazil, but the young always return to the home they were born in, always.

Mindy called me today and said there was a pair of Purple Martins on Mom's back porch. We were both shocked. Their houses are destroyed so they took up residence on a tiny chime mom had placed up high on her porch. Mindy said they take turns sitting on this chime swinging back and forth. She saw nesting material all over the porch area. They came home to Momma.

Mindy sat there and watched them soar into the sky, sing their melody and then come back to the chime to rest there in between. I think they are waiting and watching for my mother.

We always return to where we feel safe and loved and cared for.

I told Mindy to tell them, "Momma will be home soon." xoxo

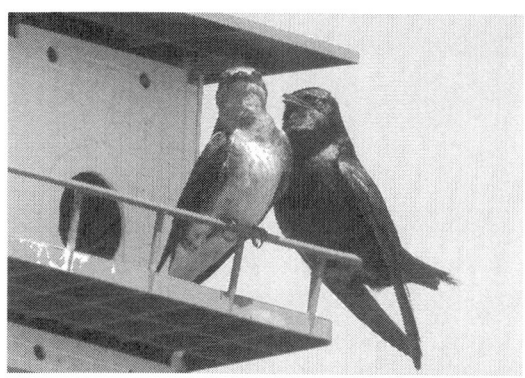

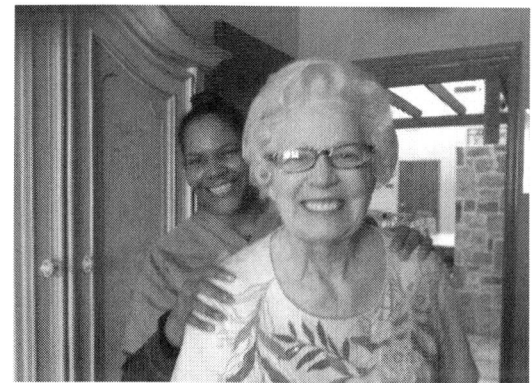

Mommy and Angeline

APRIL 25, 2013

Since Mom's illness, the last three years have been filled with more angst days than happy ones. Only lately have I felt the happier days catching up. Today was one of those monumental days. I could say all the planets were in alignment and all fell into place. But, it was not that at all. It was due to such hard work on the part of my beloved and brilliant cousin, my steadfast daughter, great professional people and the good Lord up above. Today was a day I have been promised by friends, my faith and my own convictions. Today, I saw my mom and she knew the caregiver and me by name. She also acted as though she "knew" what today all was about. It is all for you Mommy!!!!! xoxoox

APRIL 26, 2013

Patience is a virtue
Faith is a belief

Waiting is never easy
But...Justice brings relief
To those who seek truth.

APRIL 28, 2013
A lesson in humility

I spent almost five hours at Mom's yesterday. I am getting spring and summer clothes together for her. As I go through her things, I see what a truly modest person of means that she was and still is. I don't think I found one "name brand" item. My mother definitely had the money to purchase those items. The only name brand she had was Mr. Mench or Laura of Dallas. Murray's clothesline and some of these items were over twenty years old but still in perfect shape.

I found another scrapbook inside a cabinet, way at the back. It was full of newspaper clippings. More written about her as a policewoman, more cases solved. Her home is like a museum full of memorabilia of a Darby Ranger war hero, Murray, and of a pioneer policewoman, one of the first. I found some of the old yearbooks of the Dallas police department. I saw old pictures of police officers I knew as a child, teenager and an adult. I realized what an awesome childhood I had growing up in this environment around such great people. I had been surrounded by heroes and did not even realize it. I sat on the floor by the cabinet. I soaked it all up like a sponge. My mother, my mommy. Why didn't she share these things with Mindy or me?

Before I left I made one last look in her room. I looked in two more drawers. A drawer full of scarfs. I pulled out each one. I got a whiff of her smell. I took the scarf and held it close to my face. I could feel her next to me. I looked under one more scarf and there was a picture of her and Murray. There was that smile. The smile that will be embedded in my mind until the day I die. My mother's smile. The smile that says, "Every thing is going to be ok."

My mother was probably the most diffident person you would ever meet. I know there will never be a statue carved in reverence of her. If words and word of mouth could exemplify the importance of someone's life and how they contributed to society, this would be the statue I would erect in her honor.

My words I lift up to you today Mom, in honor of you.
"Call to me and I will answer you, and will tell you great and hidden things which you

have not known."
Jeremiah 33:3

APRIL 28, 2013

Mindy and I were at Mom's house today. We were doing repairs, cleaning up and carrying off old toys and so on and so on. We are putting in a new fence for her tomorrow. Mindy and I were wondering how we would ever get rid of the old swing set Bradyn and Kenady had played on for years. There was also an old spring horsey, tricycle and old toys. We were sure we would have to pay someone to do all this for us. As we were sweeping out the garage some guys in a huge truck drove down the alley and asked if we were throwing away the horsey. We said "yes" and they asked if they could have it. We said "sure" and then asked if he wanted a swing set and some other toys. He said he would love to have it. Talk about divine intervention. Thanks, God for sending that truck by today. You never cease to amaze me. You even have angels that drive trucks and pick up old toys and swing sets. Even if they weren't real angels, it felt like they were. Thanks for Your divine intervention. xoxo

APRIL 29, 2013
So full of Grace is Grace...
In the Alzheimer's community you become friends with family members of other Alzheimer's patients. You compare notes, you talk about how the person once was and you share the sadness and decline of a parent and cherished family member.

I have done this with at least four people where my mom is. Some I only knew for a month or two before they were gone, some almost a year now. It is really inspiring to see how these wonderful people had such vibrant productive lives at one time. I am beginning to think Alzheimer's is a disease that inflicts only the brightest beings in our universe.

One particular person I met from day one, her name was Grace, which suited her so well. Grace demonstrates compassion. Grace and her smile, it was the type of smile that if you turned off all the lights in a room all you would need to do is have Grace smile and the room would be full of sunshine. The first time I met her she stood up, looked at me and giggled and then smiled. At first I thought she was a visitor. Later I had the pleasure of meeting her husband, daughter and their ever-faithful dog that came to visit every afternoon.

As time went on, Grace began to decline. I would see mom trying to bandage her wounds as she sat in her wheelchair. My mother never was the "nurse" type but I am sure Grace smiled and Mom melted. There were times when they would be singing and Grace would barely be able to lift her head but I could still see her lips moving and she would still be smiling.

I can only remember once when Grace did not smile. It was the time my mom leaned over, kissed Grace's husband on top of his head and thanked him for lunch. Grace looked at mom and did not smile! We all laughed about this later. This is the world of Alzheimer's. No one bought mom lunch and I can only imagine whose head she thought she was kissing. :)

Grace, I know the angels came to pick you up Friday night. I know in my heart you are in a better place. I know how you suffered the last few months with this horrible disease. I just want to thank you for that first day when I met you. I was afraid, no; I was petrified to place my mom in a facility. When I saw you smile and make that clicking sound it was like you were saying, "This is a fun place to be and Mom would be ok." I know now that you are okay and your smile will go down in history as part of the best medicine ever administered to my mom, to Mindy and to me.
'Till we meet again. xoxoox

"Death is the opening of a more subtle life.
In the flower, it sets free the perfume; in the chrysalis,
the butterfly; in man, the soul."
- Juliette Adam

APRIL 30, 2013
A dark cloud looks menacing and carries much duress
The brain conjures up a horrible storm coming
Carries away any form of happiness
Faith carries the mighty force of winds
To push the clouds aside
And yet, the fear still lingers there at times.
Will the storm with its mighty force
Its thunder, its lightning, its hail
Follow the promises I have been given
Or take its own evil course?

A dark cloud may look like evil in its wake
May seem like the end is near
But under it is pure blue skies
Promising that indeed, that the sun will reappear.
Today the sun is shining more vividly in my life.
Thank you God!

MAY 10, 2013
Thanks Mom for giving me life so that I could be a mom...xoxo

I started thinking about Mother's Day. It is such a privilege to be a mother. A mother gives life. You share a heartbeat with her for nine months; she is your breath, your sustenance, and the life force within you. You are her and she is you for the first few months of your life and then I believe that bond goes on forever. A child's first recognition is that of sight and smell, whether it is a biological mother or an adoptive mother. A child connects with that mother's image that lasts forever and ever. Watch a baby reach its little fingers towards a mother's face or watch its eyes follow a mother around the room. Later in life a toddler reaches its hand toward a mother for comfort. If a child falls, it instinctively calls for its mommy. A mom is a nurse, a teacher, a friend, an angel, and an advocate. Moms signify life, love and acceptance.

I remember once in elementary school we had parent's day and my mom forgot the date. I was devastated. When she got home I was very upset. She worked so many hours I am sure it was an oversight. She asked me what was wrong. I was crying and told her she missed parent's day. I was so chubby and shy in those days. When my beautiful mother showed up anywhere I felt "ok" for that brief period of time, because there was this beautiful, successful woman who was my mother.

The next week while in my class my mom showed up unexpectedly. I was in shock. She asked the teacher if she could be there since she missed last week's parent's day. The teacher said yes. I can't tell you what that meant to me that day, but it meant everything.

Moms are just like that. They know when we need them the most and they make sure they are there at those times.

Thank you, Mom, for showing up that day. I wish I had thanked you more for days like that.

Thank you, Mom, for giving me life so that I would have the privilege of being a mom myself.

Happy Mother's Day.

MAY 11, 2013

Happy Mother's Day weekend to all the mommies out there, to those who have passed, those who do not have the capacity to know it is Mother's Day and to those who will soon be mommies. To all the mommies who are mommies to little animals, or to neighborhood kids, or you just mother someone, Happy Mother's Day to you too. xoxoox

MAY 14, 2013

I guess it is true; the squeaky wheel does get the oil. I have been tooting Mom's horn so much these days that I got an email from Senior Corporal of Police: Museum Curator for the Dallas Police Department to please contact him. They want to discuss Mom, and getting some of the newspaper articles from me. To be quite honest I am shocked. I felt like she should be honored and recognized for her career but it is a little like with your grandbabies, they may be the ugliest kids on the block but to you they are movie star material. To me, my mom deserves to have a movie made about her life and her accomplishments but I am her daughter and that makes me a little bit prejudiced. I think the thing that makes my mother so incredibly special is the sheer fact that she did and does not think she is anything special. She was just grateful to have a job and to help put food on our table. This is what made her one in a million. She never tooted her own horn, so maybe that is why I can't stop telling the world just how special she was and is.

P.S. If and when she ends up in the museum I will let everyone know. xoxo

MAY 15, 2013

If every thought were a word hovering over my head
Would the beautiful thoughts be flowers?
The sad thoughts, the rain?
If ideas were merely the seeds
Then there would be reason for the sadness
No flower can thrive without the rain
If I look hard enough, I can find beauty in everything...

MAY 17, 2013

I feel like a hamster on a treadmill. Run, run, run little hamster. Every day I feel so blessed that I can still remember all the tasks that need to be done in my life. Siri helps me too. I cannot imagine being one of those people who cannot remember everyday tasks. Just take a second every time you "remember" something and think of those who don't have that luxury. The mind is not only a terrible thing to waste but also a terrible thing to lose. Today I have an awesome memory by the grace of God!

"He fills my life with GOOD things".

Psalm 103:5

Pictures are the memories of yesterday...

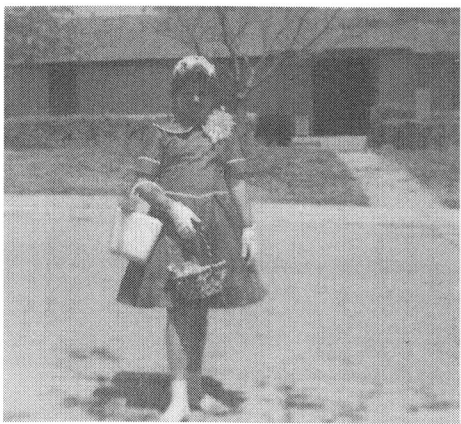

I had a pink dress it was trimmed in lace
My mother made the dress, it took many days
She cut the fabric, she pinned the pattern
I heard the sewing machine do its job
As it worked it hummed a song
My mother powered it as she pedaled along.
Clothes of mine had no name tags
Did not come in store bought bags
The only tag included in my dresses
Were the ones that would have read...
All my love,
Hand stitched by Mom with needle,
Sewing machine and thread.

MAY 20, 2013

Last night I was on overload. I had been to my mom's house. Don't get me wrong I love finding old pictures, and old notes because they prove to me how much my mom loved me. Every child, adult or otherwise, needs this. It is just the memories cause my computer brain to fill up faster than I can access the feelings. I called my stepsister, Jane. The daughter of my mom's second husband, Murray Katzen. This helped. Thanks, Jane. Later that night I called my "anchor," my father. I can just lay my heart open and tell him what is coming from my gut. All my emotions that are raw from a day of feelings, thoughts, and sentiments. I can actually feel my dad consuming some of my pain and pulling it away from me. I don't write about my dad as often as I do my mother. He is a strong man and can speak for himself; I speak for my mother because she is unable to. God has blessed me in many ways. I still have both of my parents to love and to honor. I am so blessed to have my father to call and be like a "little girl" who needs her "Daddy" when she has fallen and needs to be held to feel better. I love you Dad, thanks for always being there for me. <smoochies>

MAY 22, 2013

I can feel and see more and more each day the passing of a dark cloud that covers one's mind. It can be a cloud of real or imagined things but never the less it is real to the person feeling it. I feel as though each day I pick a new petal off this flower I hold in my hand, each petal represents a "fear" I have been holding onto. I am down to the last petals now. I can see all the petals left and the answer will be, "He loves me." God has been with me all along and He loves me!

MAY 23, 2013

Fun with Momma

Mindy, me, mom, and Nico

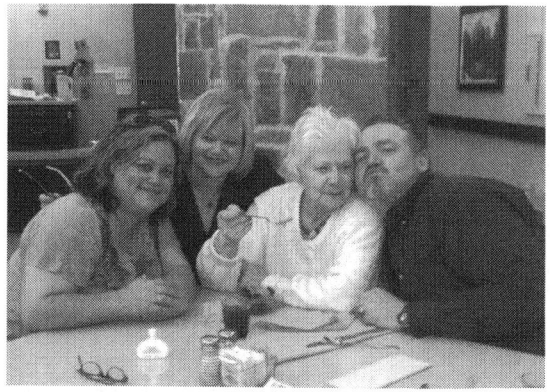

JUNE 2, 2013

My Mom has Alzheimer's...what do you do with all their clothes?

My mother's second husband had his own clothing factory, Laura of Dallas. He gave many policewomen outfits from his clothing line. My mother loved this. Many of his items were sold at Saks, and other fine stores. His factory was here in Dallas; his brand name was Mr. Mench. Some clothes in her closet have been there for over 40 years. Those with Alzheimer's don't remember from one day to the next what clothes they have, or have worn lately. They tend to think their neighbors clothes are theirs and vice versa.

You have to put your loved ones initials or their room number on their clothing. You are told in the beginning to only bring a few clothes so they do not get too confused and they can keep up with them.

I have had to go through all of her clothes, stacks and stacks of them. I pick them up and I can visualize her in them. Some I don't even remember. Some make me feel sad. Many tell a story as to when she started getting ill. I have started many stacks, only to go through them again and then change my mind. I touch them, I smell them and sometimes I hug and cradle them. A few I cry on.

When my friends have lost their parents in the past, I noticed they would keep some of their clothing for a while and quite frankly I never understood. Now I do.

Although it is only clothing, it was once next to their body. It smells of them and with me I keep thinking; she may need this when she gets well.

Of course my mom will never be "well". The facts are, her disease progresses more each day.

Her clothes are just another reminder of the dreadful disease of Alzheimer's. It robs you of even the simple things in life; including years of clothing they once wore.

God help me to get to the acceptance part. I need to let go, more for her than for me, even when it comes to the clothing she used to wear.

Mom, you are always lovely, no matter what you wear, even today. I love you.

JUNE 4, 2013

My mother has a disease that truly strengthens me. I also have the most wonderful counselor. I love you, Harry. I honestly do not know how I would have gotten through these last few years without his support. I am not ashamed to admit that I seek professional help when I need it. I believe if you can admit your weaknesses it also shows your strengths. I would say to any caregiver out there or to anyone who is suffering emotionally in any way, seek help. See your pastor, a professional or open up to a best friend you can trust. Never suffer in silence. Life is too short not to be lived and to love and to be loved. Alzheimer's is a disease in which you lose your loved one EVERY day. There is no end until the end. It is an open wound and no Band-Aid can cover it. You learn ways to keep the infection, the pain, bearable. There is no cure and we are all susceptible to getting it.

"Know how sublime a thing is to suffer and be strong".
Henry Wadsworth Longfellow

JUNE 6, 2013

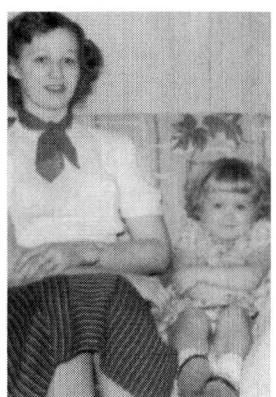

Even when I am unable to see
I feel its presence abound
It answers many questions
I am meant to look for, and some not to be easily found.
I don't sit around and question
What, who or even if it is
I just sit quietly and listen
And all the answers it gives.
That is what true faith really is.
BELIEVE...

June 8, 2013

You know the old saying, pretty is as pretty does, or she/he is so attractive but their attitude makes them ugly. I can honestly say I have never met an ugly person. I have met attractive people that I found them to become less attractive because of their attitude or less attractive people became quite beautiful to me due to their engaging smile or their gracious heart. I say this because every time I look at my mother I don't see her as an older woman. I still see her as a 30 to 40 year old person. She is also captured in that age range due to her disease. But, it is strange that "I" now see her at that age when I look at her. This only happened in the last year or so.

Because of this we are somewhat connected in her disease. This is healing to me when I see or find these younger pictures of her now. I feel her more. I feel closer to her. I feel I connect with her on a different level. Maybe it is all these knocks on my head, <smiling> never the less, it is helping me to accept losing her to Alzheimer's. I feel I am going back in time and reliving all the times we had together. The memories will always be alive through the marvelous miracle of the mind and of the pictures that captured them. My mother taught me all about beauty, not only on the outside, but the beauty inside people. That is where the true beauty of a person lies.

JUNE 10, 2013

Mindy, when you told me about this, it made my day. She has on the new blouse I just took her last week too. Yes, let's make Monday craft day. I found nine million buttons, we can surely find something to do with all of them. xoxoxo

Bradyn, Mom, and Kenady

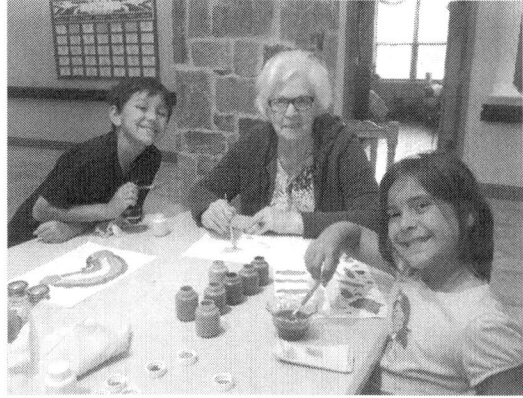

JUNE 11, 2013

Today was an exciting day, as far as alarms go. I set my mom's alarm off. I proudly put in the code, forgetting that I had forgotten the password. I was waiting for the alarm company to call me and then it hits me, I forgot the password! I called Mindy, no answer. I text her, no answer! My cell phone rings and I hear, "This is the alarm company, your alarm went off at such and such address." "Yes, I know," I answer. "It is my moms house, but I put the code in, so everything is ok. Thank you." She says, "What is the password, ma'am?" Oh shirt! I start naming every password I have ever used. She says, "Ma'am, the police are on their way, thank you!" Well, of course I look like hell because I was on my way to Tybee's for a chemical peel. My hair is on top of my head and I don't have any makeup on. I look like an ugly robber. The doorbell rings and I swear to God the most GORGEOUS cop comes to the door. He was model material. I get the third degree and he wants my identification. He can see the table inside the door and it is filled with boxes, it even looks like I have robbed the place. I am dancing around with every excuse I have. Finally, I remember I know one of police officers in my mom's town. I drop her name; "Do you know so and so?" He smiles and say, "you need to learn the password." <Whew> Now, I am either very lucky that I keep setting off these alarms or very unlucky that I keep doing it at the worst times. I am never walking out of this house again without looking like I am going to the prom. LMBO xoxo

JUNE 12, 2013

What is it about tiaras? I think every Alzheimer's patient should have a tiara for a female and a crown for a male. It takes great gallantry to fight this disease, and I bow to their courage and fortitude. xoxo

JUNE 13, 2013

I am on my way to see Mom. I will stop at Starbucks and get her a coffee and then stop and get her a sugar-free dessert. I am taking her more clothes, which they will give me the evil eye about. Now we for sure won't be able to shut her tiny closet. I decided to take her a carload of pictures too. Mindy said on Monday, when they first walked in, Mom did not know who they were. So, I am taking big pictures of all of us. Next week I am going to take cards and put names under each picture. Alzheimer's and I are going to have a tug of war. I will be damned if I give up that easily. I will do flash cards with her so she can at least remember her family. I will wear a name tag and put one on each of the kids. I don't give up easily when it comes to love. xoxoox <smoochies> I am Mary by the way.

JUNE 20, 2013

My mom's A/C unit went out yesterday. Gee Whiz. I was thinking I could shoot a little Freon in that thing and she would purr like a kitten again. No way, Jose. By the time that thing gets replaced we should be able to hook up a trailer hitch to it and pull a boat behind it. The list just keeps building on how many times she was ripped off while she was ill. As children of older parents we have to be more mindful of how others can, and unfortunately do, take advantage of them. My mother's illness caused her to lose that vitally important thing we all have inside us; that "gut feeling" that says, "NO, you are being bamboozled!" WE have to be that gut feeling for them. Elderly abuse is NEVER ok!

JUNE 24, 2013

I just got an email from two of Mom's co-workers, Patsy and Beth. I cannot say thank you enough to all those who go and visit her, especially former co-workers at the DPD. This was 32 years of her life. However, I thoroughly understand anyone who is unable to do this. Sometimes we cannot see or witness those we love suffering from an illness. It is hard to see someone who was once strong, vivacious and quick witted to not even knowing what day it is. It is hard for me to visit at times and she is my own mother. One of the many things my mother's Alzheimer's has taught me is that life is short, family is so important and love, love, love is everything. I don't have the time to tell anyone how they should feel, act or what they should be doing. My wings and halo are on back order. Xoxoxo

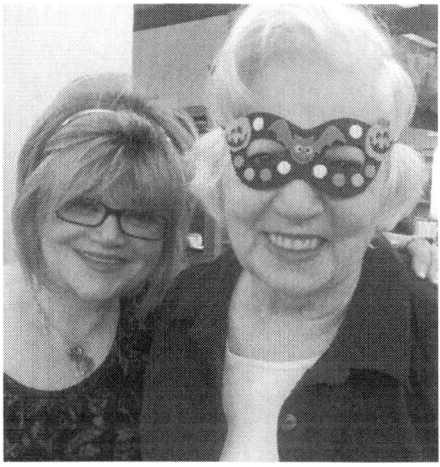

NOVEMBER 22, 2013

I got an email today from someone "Thanking" me for giving them the opportunity to meet Mom and me. Her mother passed away recently at the facility where Mom is. She went on to say that Mom was so cute and her humor always made their visits so enjoyable for her and her father. My mom has no filter now. She says what she wants and does what she wants. So, it is the real true "what you see is what you get." As time goes on I see more and more blessings and lessons learned. This is the lesson I have taken from Mom. When I see people these days, I comment on things I notice about them whether it is their hair, their eyes, or their smile; whatever I notice. I find myself touching people more. I need that contact. I see more beauty in everyone I meet, even in strangers. Maybe I have realized life is short and that we are all connected. We may have differing ideas, but we see the same moon at night, wake up to the same daybreak and we all just want to be loved, well, and kissed too. So for today I am sending out some kisses and hugs and some thanks for the wonderful people in my life and for my Facebook friends, whom I adore. xoxoxo

NOVEMBER 23, 2013

Us girls again surrounding Mom. Kenady, Mindy, me, Aunt Dot, Barbara, Tasha and mom in the middle.

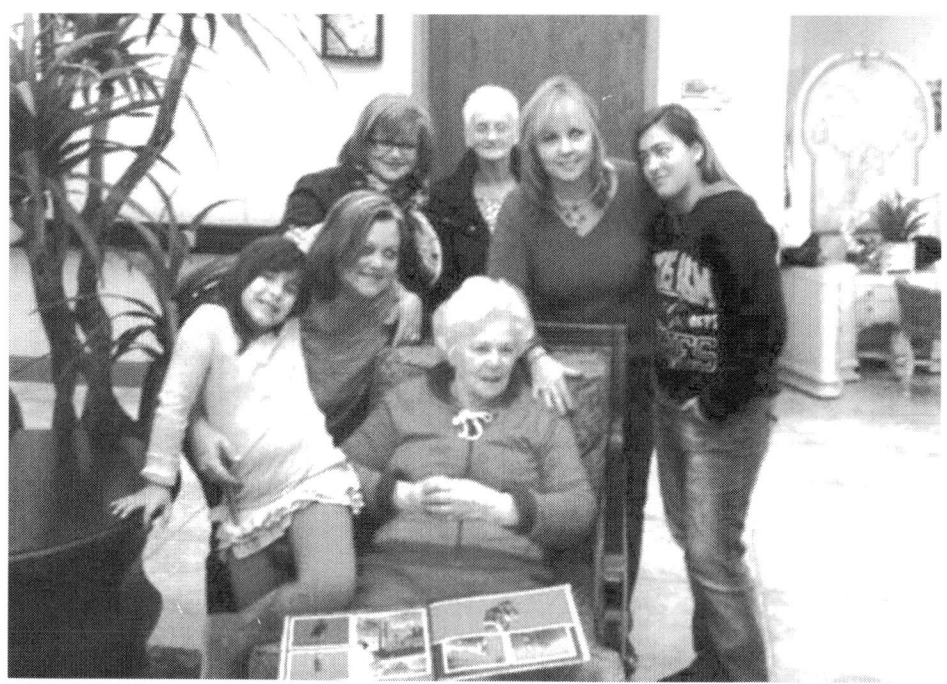

NOVEMBER 24, 2013

Each person that I meet
 has radiance inside of them
Some shine extremely bright
 and others rather dim.
It is not the words they speak
words are cheap.
Nor the fairest of them all
beauty can hide character flaws
It is deep inside the soul
the essence of man
The true contents of himself
The light emitted by ones substance

their TRUE selves, and nothing less.

Lord, let me have a light inside of me, that attracts people to me...so I may comfort and love them as I have been comforted and loved.

NOVEMBER 30, 2013

Many times I have thought about what I will name my book, my blog and the journey with my mom's illness. I am in the process of getting it ready to publish. I sit and I reflect on how to let others know what my book will be a combination of; what will the reader see and feel about my mother and me? Will it explain how I see my mother as this huge bright star that illuminated and touched everyone she met before and after the disease? A woman that helped to change things for women in the work force. Can I explain how I see her fading and the illumination disappearing, but still present in her in the midst of the disease? A star is a massive luminous sphere and in time it fades and dies. I see Alzheimer's as the fading disease. Your loved one slowly disappears, until one day they are gone. My blog/book is not a sad story. It is a story of love between a mother and daughter. A story of growth, acceptance, tears and laughter. It is a story about faith and love. It is a story about some of the brightest stars in the universe, people with Alzheimer's. The most brilliant, brightest star to me has always been my mom. So, I will name the book, "Fading Star," maybe? A blog written by the daughter of a mother with Alzheimer's xoxoxo

NOVEMBER 30, 2013

In just a few days it will be my mom's birthday. It is hard to believe it has already been a year since we gave her a surprise birthday party. I just want to thank everyone again for coming last year. I don't think she would be aware of anyone this birthday. If you came to the party, please know you were a true blessing to her and to us, her family. Happy birthday Mommy, on December 3rd. xoxoxo

DECEMBER 3, 2013

It's Mom's birthday today. Dad has surgery. I am getting my "blonde" roots done. Just another day, not! I would just like to say to them both that I am so blessed to have two of the greatest parents in the world and they still love each other even though they are no longer together. I never appreciated what awesome parents I had until I became one. I used to always tell my dad, "Dad, you were too strict on me." His answer was always, "Well, look how good you turned out!" I hate it when he uses logic on me. Thank you God for parents that loved me, but were normal everyday parents. Parents who did the best they could. I did turn out pretty ok. As Stuart Smalley would say, "I'm good enough. I'm smart enough. And doggone it, people like me."

DECEMBER 5, 2013

Got a call this morning from a loved one, it was easy to tell they were thoroughly upset. Their voice was raised, breathing was rapid and I can envision what was going on just from hearing them tell of their experience. I interrupted and said, "Take a deep breath!" They did and the change in their voice and attitude was unbelievable. I then said, this happened for a reason, now let's figure out why. By the end of the conversation we had both come to a remarkable conclusion as to why this upsetting thing happened. It was like a light went off in both of our heads. I have heard this same thing in my head over and over and over. Nothing happens in Gods world by mistake, nothing! I cannot change people, places or things. I can only change my reaction. I have to ask myself, how important is this thing to me? Is it important enough to ruin my whole day, my life? Nothing is that important. I have not always been like this that is for sure. I have learned those things in life that hurt the most are probably the best things for me in the long run. I can both learn from them and grow, or I can give up and die emotionally and spiritually. The hardest thing for me to cope with is the last few years with my mom and the events that have transpired. Some not even involving her disease. When I look at the big picture I see how all of these events have changed me for the better. I have a stronger relationship with God, a closer tie with my daughter and I think I have learned to love and accept things at face value. No one is perfect, no situation perfect. It is just the way it is supposed to be. It is out of my hands and in the hands of God. I believe, I believe! xoxoxo

DECEMBER 8, 2013

I bought my mom a beautiful pink sweater and three pairs of pants. They are so soft. I know they are too long. To save money I decided to hem them myself. I remember Home Making Class in High School when we had to make a dress. Well, I am no seam-stress and I double stitched the hem. Duh! The teacher made me an example of what not to do to a dress. I remember going home and crying. My mom could make a dress out of toilet tissue if she had to, not me. My mom went to school to speak to the teacher about this. I was so embarrassed, but my mom sat there and took up for me. She said, "I know Mary sews like a bear with gloves on, but she did the best she could." My mother rarely cried, but she had tears in her eyes that day. Needless to say the teacher never made an example of anyone who could not sew. I did learn how to hem and I am pretty darn good at it. It is a single stitch, right? Mom, I will bring you your new pants tomorrow. The bear with gloves on hemmed them for you. Grr, hear me roar. xoxo

DECEMBER 31, 2013

2013 was a blessed year for our family. I delivered some pictures of Mom, updates, and a little note to her closest neighbors, even the mail lady. She made friends with everyone. The prior years were a little hard on my daughter and myself. Our biggest answered prayer is that Mom is safe as is her estate. She is divorced, I have legal guardianship of her, Mindy, resides over her estate. Everything is back exactly the way *she wanted it*. All of mom's wishes are being fulfilled. The judicial system is a slow and winding road but it works the way it does because of our freedoms. Everyone has a right to their day in court. When we, or someone we love, have been hurt or taken advantage of we want justice quickly. I know some of the people who were part of this last year are not even on Facebook. I send you blessings by osmosis. To all my friends on Facebook who wrote while I cried and cried, I send you so much thanks and love for 2014. To my cousin, Barbara, (financial brains of family) you know how I feel about your involvement. I honestly thought at times I was going to lose it. My family, friends and my faith kept me going. This year has shown me that the guys in white hats do win. The judicial system is a GOOD thing, slow, but good. God was there all the time. When my mom awakes one day, she will see exactly how much she meant and still means to me. xoxoxoo Happy New Year, Mom!

JANUARY 3, 2014

Dear Mom...are you out there, somewhere?

Mom,

I am writing this letter to you. I don't know why. Maybe in cyber space it will find its path to you and by some miracle you can hear it.

I write this because today for the very first time you did not recognize me. I am truly sad. I am used to you getting me mixed up with Mindy but you always knew my name and that I was in the room with you. Today you did not know me.

Mom, I don't blame you for the disease you suffer with. I feel embarrassed for you because I know how important it always was for you to be in a dress or a nice pantsuit, perfectly coiffed and flawless. I never quite felt good enough to be your daughter. You seemed so perfect and yet I have learned no one is. We are fallible. Through a little girl's eyes, you were my representation of everything a woman should strive to be. So, today when I see you and you are at the mercy of a mind that has lost its way, I ask myself, *who is this woman?*

I knew the day would come when you would not recognize me. I have started forgetting what you were once like. How can a daughter say this? It looks like you, sounds like you, smells like you, and the smile is the same beautiful smile, but my mother is indeed gone.

You know what I do sometimes Mom? I talk to your pictures. My favorite pictures are the ones of you at about the age of 40. I remember you and me talking on the phone, going places with Mindy when she was little. You were so full of life then. So quick, so sharp. If I hold onto the pictures, you are still here. I can't explain it. I know you understand though.

Mom, please don't be mad at me when I cut my visits short. Sometimes when your mind is at its worst I just can't stand seeing you like that. Maybe I am a big coward, maybe I am afraid, maybe the sadness engulfs me, or all of the above.

I just want you to know, I miss you and I am so sorry you are in this mire of pure unconsciousness they have named Alzheimer's. Even if you never remember my name I will always be here. I will stay with you up until the very end. Even though I am afraid, you don't have to be. I am here.

I love you,
Mary

JANUARY 15, 2014

My mom loses more glasses than I can keep up with, or sometimes she will be wearing some I have never seen before. I gave up on prescription glasses for her. She is like me anyway, only needs them for reading purposes. I decided to get her readers but wanted to get some that were fashionable. I found a pair at the mall. They are pink and very cute on her. I wrote her name all over them; on the sides, under the lenses and anywhere I had room to write. Well, they called and said her glasses were lost. I said, "You will find them under her bed." When I got there this afternoon, the cleaning lady met me in the hall and said she had found Mom's glasses under her bed. My mom always knew MY hiding places, so, why am I surprised that I would know hers intuitively? xoxo

JANUARY 28, 2014

When I first saw my mom today, I decided the three of us needed to play beauty salon. I was the makeup artist and hairdresser. Mindy was my "assistant. In other words she kept Mom happy with the sugar-free chocolate candy. My mom loves chocolate and with chocolate we can talk her into just about anything. The apple does not fall too far from the tree. My two girls are beautiful. I am so blessed to have both of them in my life. xoxoxoox I love you Mom and Mindy. xoxo

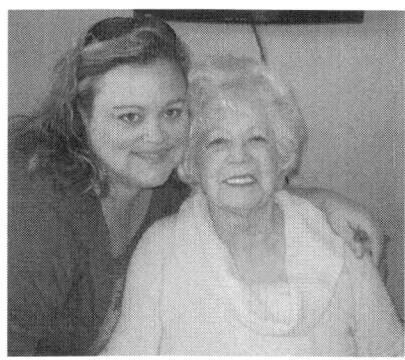

FEBRUARY 1, 2014

On my way home I stopped to see my mom. Her "boyfriend" was sitting next to her. As usual, he asked if I was her daughter. I answered, "Yes." They were holding hands. He then said in a loud voice, "I HAVE BEEN MAKING LOVE TO YOUR MOTHER!" I sat there for a minute and thought, "Oh, damn, what do I say?" I knew this was not actually happening except maybe in their minds. I smiled and said, "That is great!" They both got a big smile on their face. There was some jive music on from the 40's and I got up and danced to it. They all smiled as they sat there holding hands and chewing gum with their friend, Eloise. When I was leaving Mom said, "Mary, where is your Dad?" I answered he was at home. Just as I was walking away after kissing her goodbye her

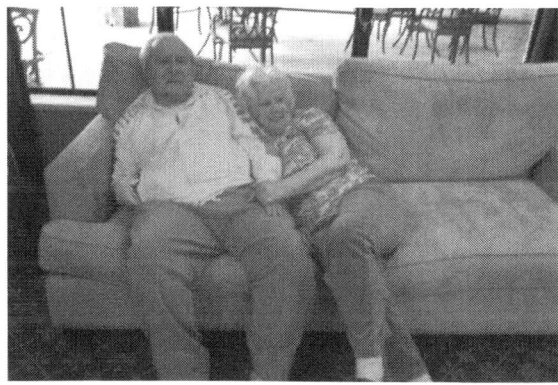

"boyfriend" said, "I hope she does not go home and tell your husband we are in love!"
I smiled and chuckled as I walked out the door. Alzheimer's is like a roller coaster ride.
I hate the hills; I wonder if the ride is going to kill me, but sometimes it can be a little
fun. I won't tell Dad, Mom, even though you are a single woman. xoxoxoo

FEBRUARY 4, 2014
The gold heart locket

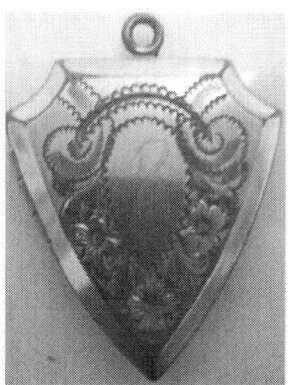

I found a gold heart at the back of the drawer
it seemed very old
I saw the engraving of an R.

Embossed with flowered etching,
no attached necklace
Just a plain piece of jewelry,
often called a locket

I examined it and noticed a clutch,
I ran my fingers across the gold trim
The heart at once released its grip
Inside were two pictures framed with-in.

It contained pictures of
two young lovers,
The pictures were small,
black and white.

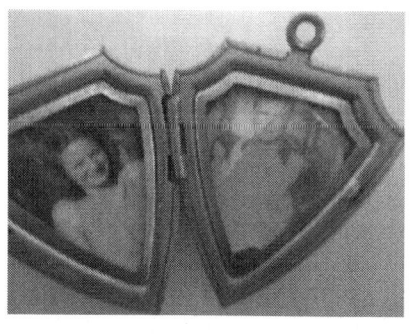

The edges were cut somewhat uneven
In the shape of a heart, smaller than a dime
As the young girl cut them, surely she
had dreams of being this man's wife.

The R was engraved with some kind of sharp
object
No fancy engraving, this was not an option
R for Rosemary, R for Ray?

Young people barely out of their teens
These were my OWN parents

Two young lovers wrapped in a dream.
When did this happen?
Why was it hidden, yet saved?

I think it was because
I was supposed to find it someday.

Many years my parents never spoke
too many harsh words exchanged
This left me feeling very alone.

Alzheimer's steals and robs
Takes away so much...
But true love always
finds its way home.

After over 40 years of not speaking to one another, my mother, asked to see my dad. They have been together two different times now. They hugged, they spoke, and there was peace between them. No longer was there hate on either side. Like I have stated before, Alzheimer's has its gifts too.

Thanks, Mom and Dad, for your love for one another, it helped to make me who I am today.

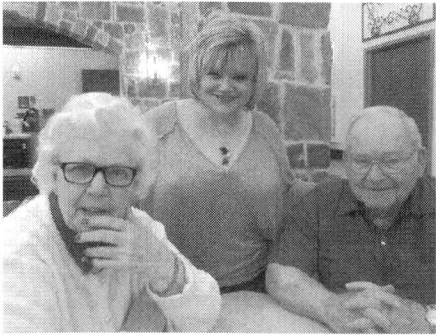

FEBRUARY 7, 2014

Tomorrow is my stepsister's birthday. I was long gone before Mom married Jane's dad and took on the job of Stepmother. Jane gave Mom and Murray a run for their money and sanity. My mom was a career woman, part- time model at Laura of Dallas, and

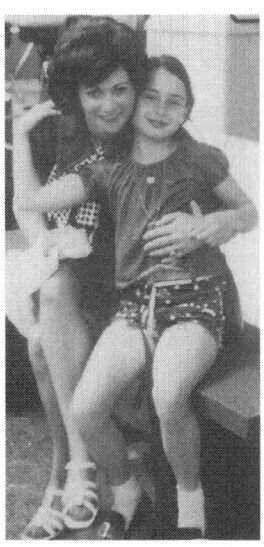

became a great mom to a cute little mischievous girl by the name of Jane Katzen. Happy Birthday tomorrow, sweet girl. Mom in her lucid moments still speaks of you. Love never ends, family is forever. Happy 40th. xoxo

FEBRUARY 10, 2014

I bought my mom a Valentine Teddy bear today holding a heart that says, "I love you." I also bought her a card. I can see her now. She will look at me, the card, and the bear and say, "Where is my candy?" Even with Alzheimer's, she still knows what is important in life. Love you, mom. xoxo

Mom loves goodies, bet you couldn't tell. LOL

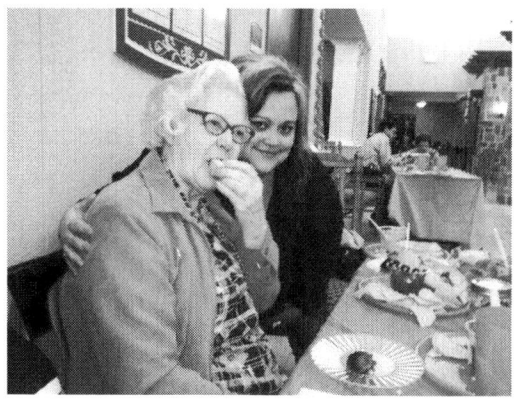

Bradyn photo bombed us! Little brat! LOL

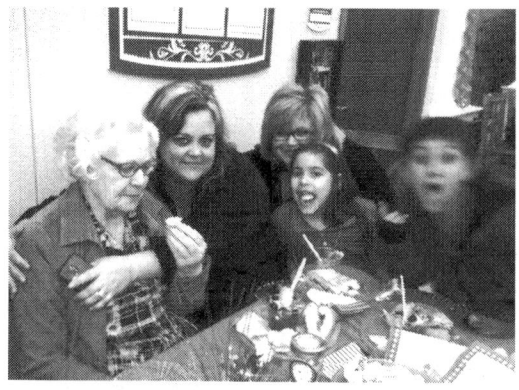

FEBRUARY 18, 2014

My mother's caregiver just text me and told me Mom was sitting next to her "boy-friend" and they were both so happy. At the Valentines party they had been sitting at opposite tables and I walked over to say "hi" to him. The first thing out of his mouth was, "Where is your mother?" They have been inseparable for months now. Who knows what goes on in their minds? I really don't care. There was an article today that came out about loneliness and it is said that it is worse on the body than being morbidly obese. This is why so many elderly people die when their spouse dies. They truly die due to loneliness. Maybe an Alzheimer patient cannot feel loneliness but who truly knows. We cannot ask them what they feel because the brain does not have an answer. If someone was once a vibrant, loving person and they find a true friend of the opposite sex to share joy with, then I say go for it! Enjoy your life no matter what age you are. My mom had two great loves in her life. She only made one bad choice when it came to love in her entire life. She loved big and was loved big. Go for the gold medal, Mom, when it comes to love. You always favored gold anyway. xoxoox

FEBRUARY 20, 2014

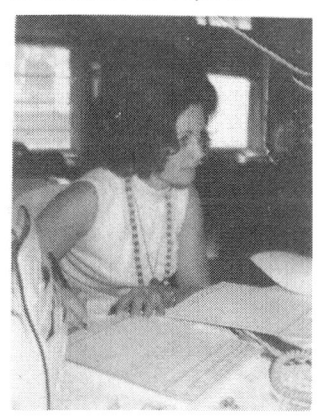 Some days I miss my mom more than others. I talked to her on the phone yesterday. She did not want to get dressed. This was the first time in almost a year I had spoken to her via phone. She did know who I was. My first inclination was to continue to talk to her like we used to; then she started telling me some outlandish story. Quickly, my excitement faded. But, honestly it was good to have someone say, "Rosie, phone for you. It is your daughter," and to have Mom say, "Oh, it's Mary?" It is not the big things with Alzheimer's I get excited over but the little bitty tiny ones. When I think of my mother, or even when I see her, I see her through the eyes of a child. She is healthy, vibrant, sharp, and always beautiful, I miss you a lot today Mom. xoxoox

FEBRUARY 22, 2014

Hey, Rocky Miele, here's a little memory poke for you. I keep running into really old pictures Mom kept. I am trying to sort them out. I thought you would enjoy seeing this picture. The couple on the left looks vaguely familiar to me and of course I can tell that is you. You sure you weren't in the Mafia? The back of the picture says 1978. Of course you can see Mom and Murray sitting to the left of you. She is smoking. I almost forgot she smoked at one time, she quit so long ago. Hope you enjoy your picture. xoxoox

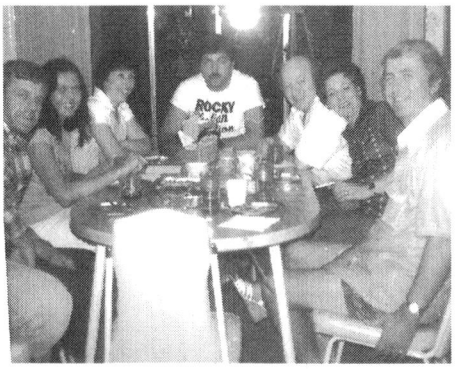

MARCH 2, 2014

Today I finished Mom's patio. I still have a few things to plant but am waiting until after the freeze tomorrow night. I want to learn how to do Calligraphy writing. I will paint "Rosemary's Garden" on the wall that overlooks the patio area. I will then take a picture and blow it up and put it on Mom's wall in her room. Because of Mindy, I also got the Purple Martin house put up and ready for her birds. All this could not have been done without Nico Friedrichs help. Sheila, Nico and I all went out to eat tonight and had a blast. Sheila, I will miss you when you leave to visit Denver. You have turned out to be a great friend to me, as you were always to my mom. Nico, again, thank you for all of your help. I think by May or June her place will look like a little piece of Heaven. It's just for you, Momma. xoxoxo

MARCH 13, 2014

I visited my mom yesterday. I always try to take her flowers and some kind of sugar-free treat. As usual she had a visitor in her room. I can always expect the room temperature to be about 80 degrees and she will be wearing socks, sandals and a sweater over her clothes. I was shocked to see she still had the ring I gave her last week and her pink glasses. Way to go Mommy! The male nurse visited while we were there to test her sugar. She adores him. Remember, I said he was MALE. She greeted him, hugged him and asked him if he was aware of how cute he was. As usual he smiled and called her "Princess." She told him she had lost her glasses and then said, "Wait, they are on my face!" We all laughed for quite some time. In fact, we laughed the whole time we were there. Upon leaving I told her I loved her and she said, "You know if you can't have some fun in this life then what's the use?" I totally agree, Mom. Even through the mire of Alzheimer's, you teach me daily acts of love and remind me of my desires to be more like you every day. Thank you, God for more days like yesterday with my beautiful mom. xoxoxoox

MARCH 17, 2014
Rocky Miele visited my mom.

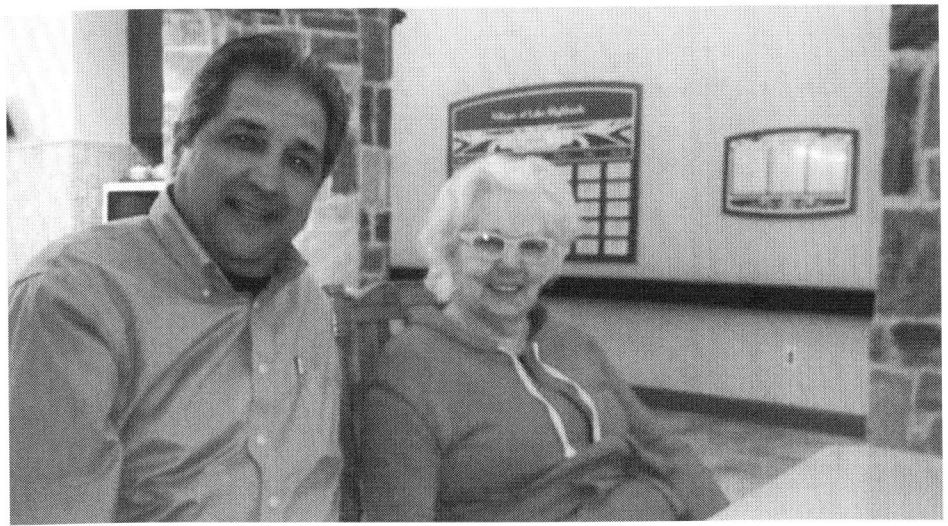

MARCH 25, 2014
I cried because I had no shoes, until I saw someone...

Lessons in life are usually learned when we lose something, or feel some sort of sorrow or pain. These are the times we can obtain knowledge about ourselves and those around us. Every time I visit my mother it is a new journey into the unknown, or a repeat lesson. A lesson where I forgot about the value of life and those around us; even those we do not personally know. They can be our teachers too. When visiting my mom yesterday, I noticed there were about five new residents. A common denominator I have noticed with Alzheimer's patients is fear; non sequential. It is hard to keep up with and much harder to understand. A person can be sitting three feet from a door and be petrified there may be no exit. There is the constant fear of wanting to go home, especially in the beginning. I can remember my mom calling me from her house and asking me to come get her and take her home. This devastated me before I had any knowledge of just exactly what her AD brain was telling her. Yesterday as we sat there, two new residents were sitting with her. One was crying and the other was saying, "I need to call my daughter. I need a ride home." This was an incessant pattern of repeating the same thought. I am very familiar with this part of the disease. I tried to change the subject each time. The lady next to her was sobbing. I told her how nice her blouse looked. It stopped her thought pattern and she smiled at me. They began asking Mom if I could take them all home and Mom said "No." I was quite surprised. The one lady asked my mother, "Don't you want your daughter to take us home?" My mom thought for a minute and said, "I don't want her to worry about us." I almost fainted. I looked at Mom and held up my hand to 'high five' her. She almost knocked me over. She is still a strong woman. We laughed. You know I realized my mom's disease has passed the "fear" mode. That was the hardest part of the disease for me. As a daughter you want to protect your parents from pain and especially from fear. I owe my mother my life. I am so grateful for days like yesterday. I felt less fear because she has less fear. It is just like my mother to make the best of things, even her disease I cried because I had no shoes, until I saw the man who had no feet. xxoxoxox

APRIL 5, 2014

My first day as Mom's dessert bakery chef. Everything must be sugar-free, low carb, and taste good. She has a tendency to ignore the word "no sweets," but with Alzheimer's the word "boundaries" is no longer a word of choice, not when it comes to cake, cookies, candy and desserts. So I have taken on the task of getting her diabetic numbers down without pumping more meds into her. Today's dessert will be a raspberry, blackberry crumble. I have to say it looks pretty bad! But, I made two and it actually taste pretty good. To be safe I am going to cover it with some sugar-free cool whip. I don't like having food thrown at me. xoxoo

APRIL 7, 2014

My mom was still in her bed at 4:00pm today. They informed me they had been unable to get her out of bed. When I walked in I pulled the covers back and opened the shades. I asked, "Mom, don't you want to get up and visit me?" She answered, "No, I want to sleep," then she pulled the covers back over her. I told her I had dessert for her and whipped cream. I saw her pull the covers off her face and she had a smile. Eventually, she got up and ate her dessert. She was down today. She was quiet. She was talking about having seen her deceased father. I had no response for her. I went into her room to clean it up. She had dinner. I came out when the dinner was finished. She was standing up pulling her sweater together that I had placed on her while she was eating. I walked over to her and she reached out to hug me. She kissed me square on the lips and hugged me for a long time. I told her I loved her. She said she loved me too. This was one of those days that I HATE this disease. There are very few days that I feel the disease wins. Unfortunately, this was one of those days. I could not wait to get home and call my dad. I knew he could, and would make me feel better. I am so grateful for my dad, Ray Birdwell. I don't think I could manage any of this without his guidance, love and courage. I am a very blessed person. I have some awesome parents and the great fortune to still have both of them in my life.

APRIL 9, 2014

Family is forever.

Mindy and mom

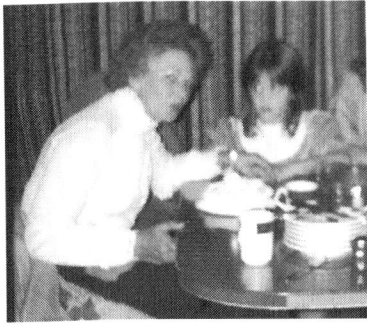

APRIL 11, 2014

I bought Mom an Alfred Dunner (on sale) purple knit sweater with foo- foo stuff at the top of it. I also got her some capris pants to go with them. I wish I could find her some really nice sandals in purple. She loves purple. I love shopping for her. I love this time of year because Ken and I go and get her Easter dress together. I would shop with Mindy but she hates to shop. They must have switched babies at the hospital. How can a kid of mine not love to shop?

APRIL 17, 2014

Another storm today, lovely. All I can think about every day when I wake up is buying another flower or bush or tree. Sometimes I wish Mom had some dirt in her room so I could plant flowers in it. The bulbs I planted are starting to come up and I planted so many at Mom's I cannot remember what they are. As they come up it is like a Christmas present, wondering what the flower will look like. I think bulbs will be my new passion. I am sincerely thinking about planting a lot more seeds and bulbs in the greenhouse and giving them away. The only thing I would ask is that when I give away a flower or bulb, people would give a small donation to the AD Association or maybe go and visit someone with AD. I would call these flowers, "Gifts From Rosemary's Garden." It would be my chance to share my love of gardening and to remember that as the flower grows, so does our hope for a cure. xoxoo

APRIL 17, 2014

Got a surprise visit from a dear friend today, Angeline. She was one of mom's favorite caregivers. Mom was in an awesome mood. She kept telling everyone how beautiful they were. Even the males were pretty and we laughed and laughed. Thank you LORD for laughter!

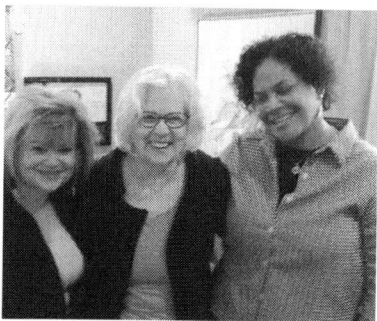

MAY 2, 2014

I saw my mom yesterday. Again, I had to get her out of bed. This time I used yogurt, diet cherry limeade, and last but not least, a sugar-free, chocolate covered marshmallow. If all else fails pull out some chocolate. Upon rising, I noticed she had on two different sandals. She wears a size 7. Not only was the shoe not her shoe, not on the right foot, but also it was a 9 1/2. Her socks also said a different room number. I looked in her drawer, she had tons of socks. Now I had to find her other shoe. I searched under her bed and found a silver slipper, not hers. OMG. I did finally find the match to the 9 1/2 shoe and the match to her other sandal. I took it to the front. I also found a pair I had totally forgotten about. Mom and her shoes. She had a thing for shoes. I took the match out to her, rubbed her feet for a minute and then put her shoe on. I said, "Now, doesn't that feel much better?" She asked, "What?" These are the times I giggle and she will ask me what is so funny. Then we both laugh. xoxoxo

MAY 5, 2014

It has been an emotional weekend. I read in a caregiver pamphlet that we must remember through all trials and tribulations that God says, "It came to pass." I remember as a teenager being so afraid of a test or an essay in front of the class that I would worry myself into frenzy. As an adult, I worry all night about a medical diagnostic test for the following day. After these events were over I said to myself *that was not so bad, I lived through it.* Some days are harder than others when it comes to emotions, events, and when I think I can't do this or that for another day. But I do, and I grow from the day's events. I find I don't have to be alone and that God always puts someone in my life that gives me the exact answer I need. I don't think I go one day without someone telling me they love me. How precious is that? Lord, help me to always tell someone, anyone who is hurting, that I love them just when they need to feel and hear it. xoxo

MAY 6, 2014

To all those who visit my mom, she has been moved to a different unit. She is in the same facility but now she is in the 800 unit. You can go to the nurse's station in that unit and ask for her room. This is a bigger unit with more nurses and aids. She will have better care and be around more people. Today when I visited her she seemed down. I knew exactly what to do. I told her I bought her a new blouse for a dollar at a garage sale. Love lie #1! I got it at Macy's but she loved it even more because she thought I only paid a dollar for it. I told her I brought her 'homemade' brownies that were not sugar-free. Love lie #2! She said, "Oh boy, oh boy!" I showed her some red fingernail polish and told her I would paint everyone's nails there but she would be first! Love lie #3! I only painted hers. By the time she had her brownie, a hamburger, saw her new purple, flowered, one-dollar blouse, and got her fingernails and toenails painted, she was no longer sad. Upon leaving she looked at me and held my face between her hands. She said, "Mary, I really miss you." I said, "Mom, don't make me cry." My mom and I have never been closer and yet so far apart. I cherish this time of love between us. Those times are real and I will always remember the truest love we shared through the mire of Alzheimer's. Thank you, God for knowing exactly what I need. xoxo

MAY 11, 2014

We can't seem to talk Mom into going anywhere these days. So we just take ourselves to her. I really wanted her to see her garden. Maybe next time. We all layed in the bed with her and cuddled. She seemed tired today but she was so glad to see us. Sometimes she seems to think Mindy is the younger me and I am the older me. Kenady seems to be the "little Mindy." Whatever works for Mom, works for all of us. We all loved spending time in the bed with you today, Mom. I love you.

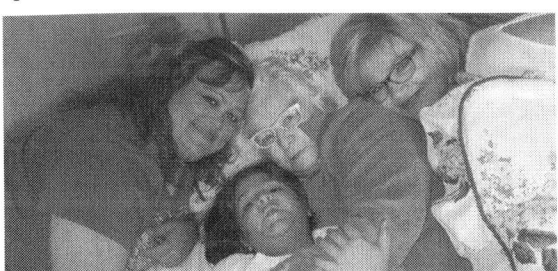

MAY 13, 2014

Got a call last night about my mom. My irrational fear went from 1 to 90 in about a ten second time frame. The first call I make is to my rational daughter. At first, I am somewhat calm and last about 60 seconds. Then fear takes hold and the tears come. My daughter reassures me and says everything will be ok. I feel better and I can feel some realm of calmness and rationale. The nurse calls me back and I trust him implacably. I feel my body relax more. At times I am totally unable to find my way. These are the times I see how God works through others. A conversation on Facebook with a friend, a call to my daughter, a text from a friend. These are not happenstance. I don't have all the answers, but I am blessed to have friends and family who do. xoxoox

MAY 21, 2014

I think I will have a whole chapter in my book called, "The Best Laid Plans." Just because you think something is one way does not necessarily make it so. Case in point: As stated before my mother loves purple. I spend hours searching the stores for purple clothing. Try it sometime; there are not a lot of purple items. I found a purple, Alfred Dunner sweater that was extremely expensive. I talked myself out of buying it. Each time I went into Macy's it would be at a lower price. I went in a few days ago and it was down 50%, plus I had a coupon. It was mine. Mom will love this. It is purple, soft, lightweight, has little tiny sequins, it was awesome. It even had a camisole and a necklace that went with it. I cannot wait to see her face when I give it to her. Yay! When I walked in yesterday afternoon, she was lying in bed. I tapped her. "Mom, wake up I have something for you!" She slowly turns and looks at me. "I am tired," she says. "But Mom, look what I brought you, a purple sweater with sequins!" She looked at the sweater and looked at me. She said, "I don't like it." Then she went on to say she did not like my blouse either. It was a day when I knew she did not feel well. I don't stay long on these days. I know when it is not a good time for her. Upon leaving I asked her if I could hug her. She said, "Sure." I gave her a long hug, kissed her and started to walk out. She said, "You can leave the sweater, I MIGHT wear it some time." I smiled to myself. I am sure she will love it tomorrow! xoxoo

MAY 23, 2014

Remember the purple sweater my mom said she did not like? Well, yesterday I got a text from my mom's favorite nurse where she resides. His name is Obie and I'm pretty sure she has a crush on him. In the afternoon, the only way he can get her to eat is to tell her she needs to get up so he can come by and take her to dinner. She promptly rises! In the text was a picture of her. She had on the whole ensemble I had gotten her. I did not pick out the socks but they did have purple in them. Heaven has a special place for nurses like Obie. xoxo

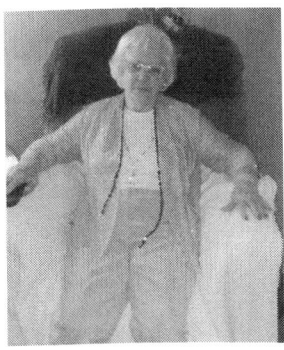

MAY 25, 2014

I have seen my mom more often recently as she is having more difficulties psychologically. I walked in yesterday and finally found her in the corner of the entertainment room. She was talking to the med nurse and was all bundled up and shivering. Her teeth were even chattering. I asked as I walked up if she was cold. She promptly looked sternly at me and asked, "Who are you?" I said, "I am your daughter silly" and I smiled. She replied sternly again. "You are not my daughter!" Normally this would make me cry. This time I looked straight in her eyes and said, "I damn sure am!" She did not say another word. I told her I was going to get her another blanket. When I returned, Addie was checking her sugar. I covered her with her purple blanket, she was still shivering. I decided to get on the chair with her and completely cover her body. I wrapped my arms around her and told her I would warm her up. I am sure we looked ridiculous. Mom looked at the med nurse and asked her if her kids did this to her? She smiled and told my mom, "Yes." After a few minutes she seemed to warm up and I removed myself and just rubbed her arms and legs. It was time for dinner. I took her to the table, blankets and all. I kissed her goodbye. As I walked away I heard her say to the group at the table. That was my baby. xoxo

JUNE 10, 2014

I visited my mom yesterday afternoon. I was feeling pretty happy after seeing Tybee. I have some awesome friends who charge my battery. Mom has a new friend by the name of Betty. Betty repeats everything over and over again. A stage mom went through herself. She is much more engaged than Mom is. I am by no means a doctor, but I do know my mother, and I would guess we are sliding into third base. The third part of the disease. The last stage. I took her the usual sugar-free goodies and flowers and sat to talk to her. Her friend Betty always tells Mom how much she loves her and I call Mom Marilyn Monroe now. I love her platinum hair and the way they fix it. There was a gentleman sitting at the table. Betty leaned over and asked him if he was married to either of them. He did not reply. She looked at me very intently and for the umpteenth time asked me if I was indeed "this lovely woman's daughter whom she adored." I answered, "Yes" like it was the first time she had asked. She said, "Honey, it is no fun getting old. Do you have a husband or a boyfriend?" Before I could even answer she began to tell me to have lots of sex. She explained to me that one day I would be too old to do it and I should do it every day. She then begins to get really graphic and I burst out laughing. We all had a big laugh. I thought it was time for me to exit. Those that have Alzheimer's have no filter and sometimes I think that is great. They are just like children, they say exactly what they see or feel. On the way out I told Betty I would get back to her.

Thanks God, for putting Betty in Mom's life. xoxox

JUNE 20, 2014

Today she thinks I am Mindy. I did her nails and she loved the flowers out of her garden. Doesn't she look cute in jammies? xoxo

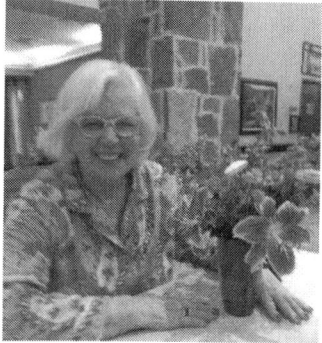

JUNE 25, 2014

Mom told me on Tuesday (I had worn my hair curly) that she liked it straight and not curly. As soon as she saw me yesterday, my hair was straight, she said, "I don't like your hair straight, I like it curly." xoxo

JUNE 26, 2014

I have the most awesome Son-in-Law, Tony Stevens. Mindy was unable to attend a program with me at Mom's facility on Thursday night, Tony, who is always extremely busy, gave me an immediate "Yes" when I asked if he could bring the kids and meet me to see Mom. He is such a wonderful father to my two grandbabies, an awesome husband to my daughter and is always kind to me. I want to personally thank him for making it easier on me and much more fun for Mom.

Kenady, Tony, Bradyn, and Mom

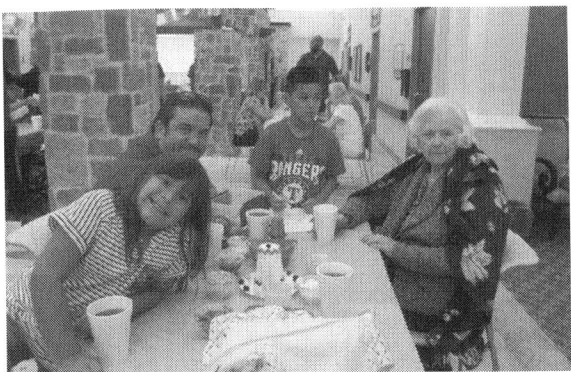

JUNE 27, 2014

On the way to my mom's yesterday I could feel myself getting sad. All these negative thoughts going through my head. The "poor me," "I can't do this forever," "This is so hard to do." Earlier that day I had picked up Dolly's new CD. I am not even a big fan, although I love her humor and the way she can laugh at herself. So, I purchased the CD. Of course the first song on there was this one. The words are so true. It's the same old adage; the more we give to others the more we receive. God is always with me, always! Have a great weekend everyone! xoxo

JULY 1, 2014

I feel such elation, exultant gladness, at this moment. The podiatrist just called and told me she had cut moms toe nails and worked on two of her toes that looked somewhat suspicious. Why would one think something so easy and insignificant for the average normal person to perform, cutting ones nails, could cause such joy? As we grow older, and if we suffer from any disease, these tiny tasks can become insurmountable, almost impossible. So, we depend on others to undertake these tasks. I try and perform these types of tasks for her but I am not a doctor. My mom depends on nurses, caregivers, aids, and last but not least, family. It is all a full circle, even down to cutting toenails. I feel such JOY when I allow myself to receive help and blessings from others, even little things. xoxo

JULY 3, 2014

Mindy went to see Mom today. The aids handed Mindy a framed picture. The same one

I sometimes find in Mom's bed next to her. I usually place it back on her nightstand. It is a picture of her and Murray Katzen, her deceased husband as of 2000. Mom truly loved my father but sometimes people grow apart over time. I truly believe Murray was the love of her life. He gave her peace of mind and less concern about some of her biggest fears in life. She was blessed to be loved by two wonderful men. Yesterday, she walked around the facility with her framed picture telling everyone this was her husband and she was his wife. It was a good day for her yesterday. As I have stated before, Alzheimer's may rob the mind but the heart never forgets love.

And now these three remain: faith, hope and love. But the greatest of these is love. One day Mom, one day. xoxoxo

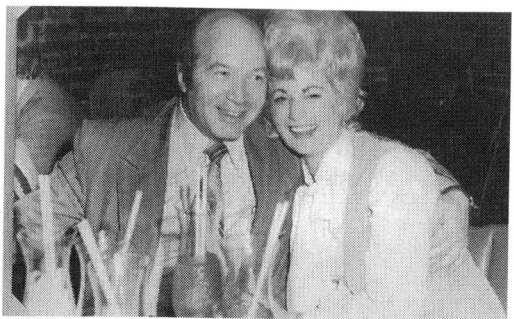

JULY 7, 2014

We were trying to kiss but our noses got in the way.

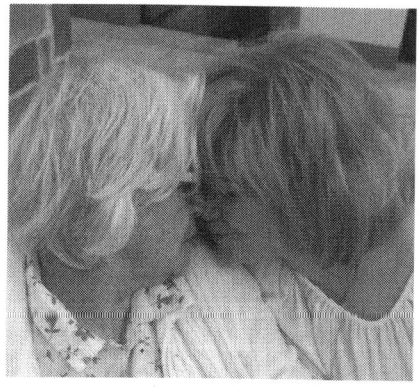

JULY 12, 2014

My mother was never much of the kissing type before AD. Now, she wants to kiss all the time. There are blessings in most everything if you just look for them. Sometimes you may need a magnifying glass. But, they are there. Thank you God for giving me a magnifying glass mind.

JULY 16, 2014

I got a call a few hours ago. It was about my mom. She, I mean her brain, I have to learn how to separate the two, were having some problems today. The Alzheimer's brain does such marvelous things your parent would normally not do. It took me a while to realize it was not her fault, nor mine, nor God's. So, I took a deep breath and we discussed a plan and I will go there tomorrow and take her some more sugar-free chocolate chip cookies. Thank you God for cookies. Anyway, I digress. I started thinking that one day I too will be old and maybe I will do some weird things, worse than now. But anyway, I came up with this silly poem about getting older. We should take the responsibility of loving and caring for our older parents. It is not a choice in my opinion, it is a gift and we can find the time. xoxoxo

We are the masterpiece of our parents love

Age...it's just a phase

Puberty same as old age

You get a zit at fifteen

A few wrinkles at fifty

Both look better after

You cover with gooey plaster (makeup)

Some things better when you're younger

You get away with more when you're older

That makes it even more fun...

Do I wanna get old

Hmmm, let me think for a minute,

Hell no!

God, if you are reading this, I don't want to die either, so I will take getting older.

JULY 22, 2014

If you want a real treat then go to a memory care unit. If you want to be enlightened, then visit a nursing home and sit with a group of senior citizens. It is almost like opening a book and reading about each person in the room. You can tell so much about a person by their dialect, their proper use of the English language, their use of words, people they discuss, their humor, their demeanor. Even through the mire of Alzheimer's they are still there. Their history comes out in different flavors. It may be disjointed and repeated, but like a puzzle, if you sit and listen you can put it together and find the history of a once great mind. I have found that the elderly are not washed up individuals. They are actually wise, prophetic, warm people who are open to discussing sex, fun, family, and laughter. They too were young once. If only we could get past our fear of becoming old I think we could appreciate them for what they truly are. Treasures, all of them, like fine antiques that only grow more priceless as time goes on. xoxoxo

Brighter than the stars of Heaven,
Brighter than the dazzling sun,
We shall shine among the ransomed,
When our work on earth is done.
"Saints Reward" by William G. Schell

AUGUST 1, 2014

Have you ever noticed that everyone has their own distinct odor? You can walk into any home and it is there. I am not talking about perfume, but every person has their own body odor, his or her personal scent. When Mindy used to stay the night with her Nana, my mom, I would open her overnight bag and I could smell exactly where she had been. I went to visit Mom today and decided to change her sheets. I noticed it had been a while since her bedspread had been washed. She loves that bedspread. It is white with ruffles along the edge and it has purple flowers all over it. I placed it in a plastic bag and brought it home. I realized just a few minutes ago it was on the floor in the laundry room. As I tore open the bag it was like my mom popped out of the bag. I could smell her like she was standing right next to me. The spread is full of stuffing and it is big and fluffy. I just grabbed it for a minute and held it to me. I could pick that smell out of a million other smells; that is my mommy. Bradyn, my grandbaby, is so bonded to Tony, his dad, but when he is hurt or afraid he wants his mommy. Moms are a wonderful thing and even better when they smell yummy. xoxoxoo

AUGUST 2, 2014

Thank you to Lisa, Rocky and Cleo for visiting mom today. I am sure she was so glad to see her cherished neighbors. People tend to forget those who are in facilities.

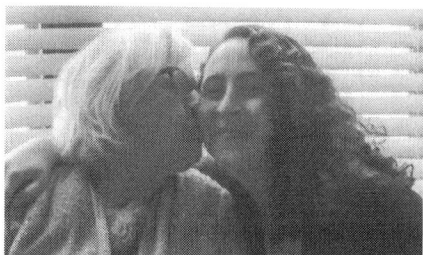 It could be due to many factors and I understand, but those who do remember are very, very special people. May God bless you for taking time out of your day to bless her with your love. She and Murray loved everyone they ever came in contact with. I am sure Murray was right there with you guys today.

AUGUST 12, 2014

I saw my mommy last night. She was sitting at the dinner table sound asleep. I lightly ran my finger across her hand and she looked up. Her hair has never been as long as it is now. It is not actually white it is more platinum blonde. It is beautiful and soft and lovely. I looked at this woman that is going to be 80 years old in December. She has fewer wrinkles now than she did ten years ago. No worries equals no wrinkles, I am guessing. I gave her sugar-free chocolate graham cracker cookies. She was super happy. Obie, my favorite nurse, came over and she was immediately overjoyed. He asked her who was visiting her and she looked at me with a question mark on her face. She said, "I don't know?" He said, "That is your daughter." She said, "Oh, Mindy?" Well, she got close. I later walked with her to her room. She is getting closer and closer to needing a walker. We already have a red one with a seat and it is very trendy. Can a walker be trendy? I know she doesn't know what is going on, but every time I leave I feel for her. I transfer my sadness into her mind. I imagine how she should be thinking. Projection has always gotten me into trouble.

"Do not be afraid; do not be discouraged." -Deuteronomy 1:21

AUGUST 17, 2014

God has a plan for everything we do. Many times I wonder just exactly what His plan is for me as a caregiver. Of course there are those days that the light of knowledge goes off in my head and I have a distinct revelation. There are also those days I want to scream at the heaven's and ask "Why me? Why my mother?" I often ask God how much longer I have to watch my mother suffer. Do I have to watch her lose all of her capacities, every one of them? Is there some special lesson here? If so, I don't want to be a good student at times. I want to skip school, run away. Would God give up on me? Never! The precious daughter that God gave to me many years ago helps me through another tough day, worse than most. God will send to me the necessary encouragement. Most times if I help another, it will intuitively help me more. I pray in some small way I am helping someone else who also has questions at timesxoxo

"Lord, you have assigned me my portion and my cup; you have made my lot secure" -Psalm 16:5 NIV

AUGUST 21, 2014

Tending my mother's garden has taught me so much. I have learned more in the last year about her, about myself, about loss and also about new life. I believe her essence is in and around her garden. I have fought so many battles with so many plant diseases and actually won. Many of her fruit trees, flowering bushes, and vines were on their deathbed, and through my tenacity they are all thriving. I decided I would not let one more thing be diseased that had to do with her. If I could not make her well, I would make everything around her progressively better. In the spring I purchased a passion vine for my mom's garden. I had the hardest time finding one. After finding one at a specialty garden I remember the clerk saying, "It is a pretty vine if you can stand the worms that get on it!" I was thinking EWW, worms? I did not care; I was on a mission to fulfill my dream of replacing all of mom's flowers and vines. I kept watching for those "worms". A few months past and lo and behold, one day in August I saw the tiniest of worms. It was so little but over the next few days, after gobbling up much of the passion vine's leaves, it was huge. I wanted to dispose of it but instead I looked it up online and realized it was going to become a butterfly. I have had so much joy watching those "worms" turn into butterflies week after week. I often wonder why the clerk did not say that the plant would be covered with caterpillars and butterflies and I would get so much enjoyment out of seeing them in the garden. I think that is how I am at times with my mother's disease. I get so upset each time I see her and she has regressed. I get depressed and I cry and feel so sad. That is not the acceptance I have promised God I would try and have.

As I watched her eat a hamburger the other day, she took her onion and her sugar-free cookie and she spread the icing on the onion. At first I wanted to say, "No, Mom, the icing does not go on the onion," and then I looked around the room and there were some who could not even feed themselves. So, I saw the butterfly and not the worm. OK, it is a weird analogy. But, it goes to show how we sometimes see things. Who knows, icing might be pretty good on a grilled onion! Who am I to judge? As long as Mom can pick up her food, then today, I am pretty sure I will be grateful.
Lord, please let my love for others who are caretaking cover them like a warm blanket when they need my encouragement. xoxoo

Mom and her long hair, my 'look alike' Marilyn Monroe, Mom. I have never in my entire life seen her hair this long, EVER.

Mom and John

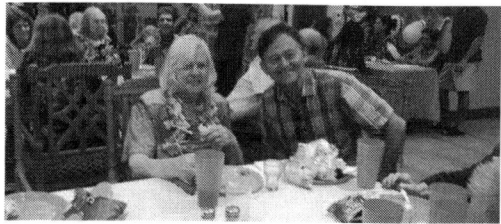

AUGUST 28, 2014

It is so hard to explain the relationship between a grandparent and a grandchild. When I was younger, I would wonder how my mother could somehow show my daughter more patience, more tolerance and at times more love than I suspected she had me. I had to become a grandparent to understand the love you have for your grandchildren. It is unique in every way. It's like the creamiest icing on the moistest, most delicious cake. The cake can be oh so yummy, but the icing is the crown for the delicious cake. Grandbabies are the dreamiest and the creamiest! The stroke of grace. Today when visiting my mother she was again only using disjointed sentences, mumbling at times. We brought her cookies and a sugar-free lemon pie. She can barely hold a fork now and sits in a wheelchair. She has definitely had a dip in her AD. I left to go to her room. While changing her sheets my daughter walked in. She had the saddest look on her face. She expressed to me that Nana had told her she could not put socks on her because she did not know who she was. She said, "Mom, she has never said that to me before." I knew my daughter was extremely sad. We straightened Mom's room and then went out to say goodbye. Nana (Mom) kissed us both goodbye and mumbled something. I did not say much about it then, but would like to tell my daughter now. Your Nana loved you more than anyone and at any time. She was able to love you totally without any conditions. She loved you without any fear of being abandoned or judged. It is just that way with grandparents. We love unconditionally and for some reason our grandbabies see us only as their hero's. She will always know who you are in her "heart" if not in her diseased mind. You were and are her pride and joy. I promise. xoxoox

SEPTEMBER 7, 2014

To all those who have sent me the Alzheimer's video of the mother and daughter lying in bed, I want to sincerely thank you. The video reminds me of so many times I have done the same thing with my own mom. My mom's disease is progressing and we have a tough time communicating now. She does not eat as well as she once did and she does not quite follow any conversation. But, we do the best we can. You know the old saying, it is quality not quantity. In the case of AD, a minute is worth a day sometimes. I receive so much love from others it fills that empty spot. Knowing that others are following my journey and care about my mom and me is very healing. Thank you for loving my mom and me. Xoxoxo

SEPTEMBER 18, 2014

My mom with some of her comrades at the DPD. They were under cover at the time and in street clothes. I am not even sure who the other guys are. I wish I could find a retired police officer to name them for me. The smile on moms face is how I will always remember her and how beautiful she is. That is how I see her, even now.

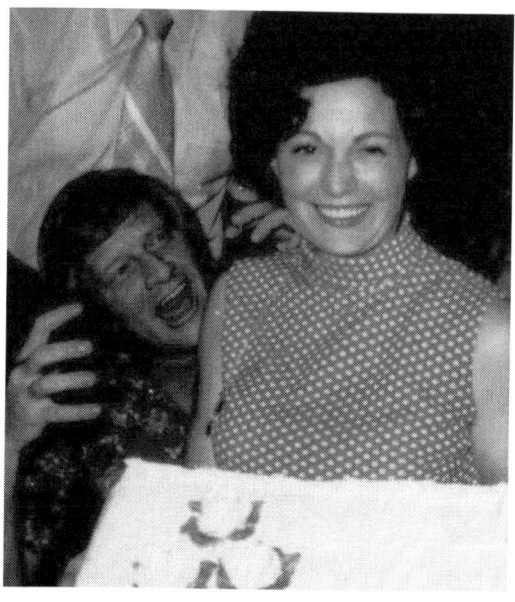

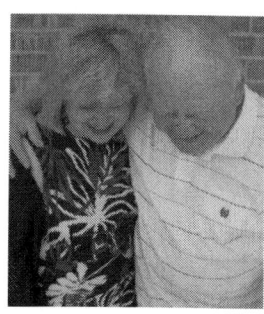

SEPTEMBER 20, 2014

I write about my mom and her illness quite frequently. My dad always makes me laugh, is always there for me when I cry and always tells me the truth about my literary talents. Quite frankly, I don't know what I would do without him and if he knows what is good for him, he will live to be 100 OR older. <smoochies for you Dad>

SEPTEMBER 23, 2014

I was looking on my calendar today as I was finishing my annual guardianship papers for the court. It has been almost two and a half years now that mom has been safe and in sole care of Mindy and me. I think the brain has a way of allowing bad memories to go to the back of the line. I could have sworn it had been years longer. I will never forget February of 2010 when Mom was lost. You don't hand keys to someone with AD and expect them to follow you somewhere in a car. If I let my mind remember all the "what ifs," it would surely destroy me. So, I will allow myself just today to remember the horrific trials we went through. I will then put it all at the back of the line, so to speak. Where did I get the strength to do what I did during that time? My only answer is that it came from God. My mom is safe, well fed, and so thoroughly loved. I pray for all those in this world who are exploited, abused or taken advantage of in ANY way. I always said, we needed a hero in mom's case. It just so happened there were many of those. Thank you God for the past, and let it stay there. I pray for anyone who is in need, to be delivered their own hero at this time.

"If we endure, we will also reign with him" -2 Timothy 2:12

SEPTEMBER 26, 2014

Today I am, taking Mom a bunch of goodies. She gets a purple scarf, purple top, purple socks and some warm, snuggly house shoes. The trim on the shoes has some purple in them too. I put her name on everything but if something gets misplaced and it is purple, they immediately know whom it belongs to. All these things and some sugar-free chocolate chip cookies. The funny thing is that she will not care about the clothes or shoes; it will all be about those cookies. That smile on her face when she sees those cookies makes me happy the whole day. Thank you, God for chocolate in all its forms. Have a great weekend beautiful people. xoxoxo

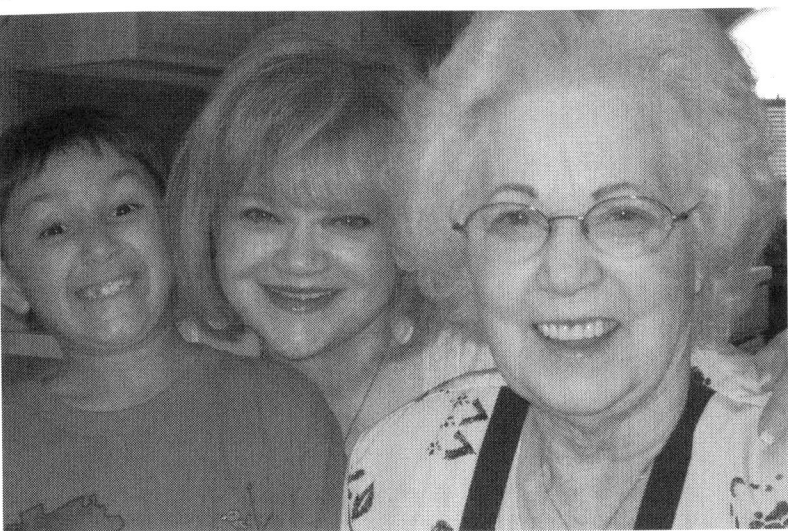

OCTOBER 8, 2014

I never knew just how good she was doing when this picture was taken, until I saw how much worse she could get. You live and learn with this disease. She does not know us anymore and I stopped knowing her long ago. I still "feel" that she is and was, and will for forever. I love you, Mom. Mindy and I are still here for you, always.

OCTOBER 16, 2014

Mindy said, "C'mon Nana, let's take a selfie". She asked her if she knew who she was. She said, "I am not sure, I am sure you are someone I love."

Mom and my daughter Mindy

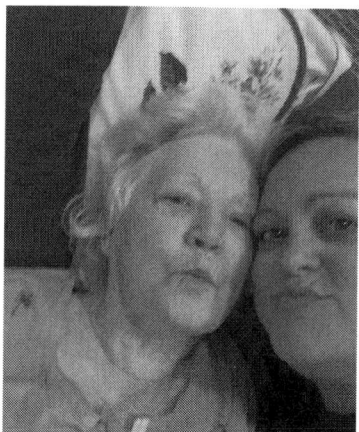

October 17, 2014

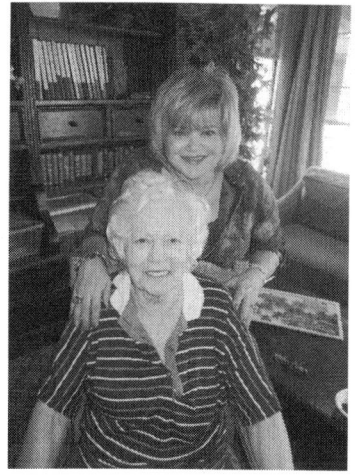

Acceptance does not mean you like it...
She knew me last week, but not today...
I feel quiet numb as she looks through me
and then looks away.
"Mom, mom...do you know who I am?"
That look answers my question
 when she can't...
I visit with this stranger, this faded image
of what once was
I've long missed missing her...
 I have acceptance of
The inevitable.
I know that is what she wants from me,
Mindy, all of us.
All of those who love her.
I'm working on my acceptance Mom, I promise.
10/17/14

My all-time favorite pic of you and Mom. You have truly been a blessing to our family

My mom and Nico.

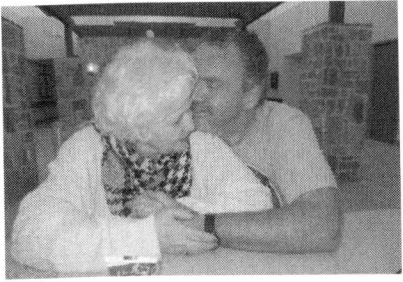

OCTOBER 21, 2014

Letting go and Letting God
Letting go when you want to hold on
 is never easy.
I beg "Don't go, PLEASE"...
And the spirit whispers
"Let me, It is time to leave"
I stayed as long as you needed me.
"I still need you!" and the spirit cries
"If I go now, I will leave with dignity"
Letting go is self-less, with her, I tend to be selfish.
"Just a little more time please!"
Maybe months, or just a day or two,
And the spirit smiles-
Just as I knew it would.
10/20/14

OCTOBER 30, 2014

I remember my parents dressing up for one Halloween. In those days there were no store bought costumes and a Trick or Treat bag was actually a bag, paper sack or a pillowcase. I wish I had time to find this one picture of them. They both had a stocking on each of their heads. I bet my dad still remembers this. They looked ridiculous and yet so funny. My parents were always happy and so much in love. It was just the three of us. I have so many good memories of every holiday with them. My parents were not perfect while I was growing up, but I am quite sure I was not the perfect child either. I hope everyone has a safe and memory packed Halloween. Much Love. xooxoxo

NOVEMBER 1, 2014

Well, today was a new chapter for our family concerning my mom's Alzheimer's. We brought in Hospice to take over her care. It was an insightful day for me today. There were tears and new insights. I felt some freedom for her and less guilt for myself. I want my mom to have dignity in her final days, months or years. Whatever God has in store for our journey left. I will not be posting any more pictures of her. I got this feeling the other day that she might not want others to see her decline and so I will only post our journey and pictures of her garden and former pictures of her. I want to thank Hospice for the most kind RN they sent to visit with me. Of all things she is a writer like me. God knows just what I need when I need it. He always has. You are in good hands, Mommy. xooxox

NOVEMBER 4, 2014

I went to pick up some papers this afternoon about Mom. I always feel better if I buy her something. Heck, I feel better if I buy anyone something. I probably get that from my mom. She was not a big spender but she still bought people things. She saved every penny she made. She loved to buy me presents on Christmas but I never had to wait until Christmas morning to open them. She always found some excuse to give them to me early. Some of her excuses were as follows: Santa came early to our house, I was especially good that year, she had to work the midnight shift so Santa had to come early so she could see me open my presents, etc. So, what do I do now? The same silly thing I make up other excuses. So, tonight I bought her some purple pajamas, some purple house shoes, some flowered pajamas, a scarf and I got me a new coat. I will pretend my mom got it for me way before Christmas. She would like that! xoxo

NOVEMBER 15, 2014

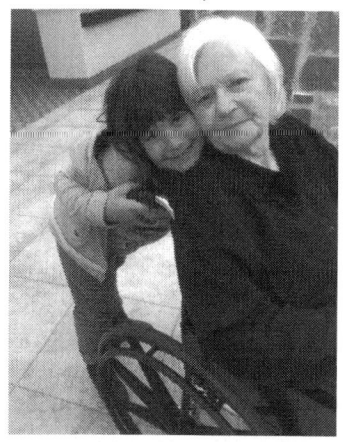

I hobbled in to see my mom today. I had tripped over some firewood next to my back door and fell right on my knee. I had to wear a "cast" for six weeks. It was a long distance to get to my mom's room on crutches. Kenady was visiting her. They were both holding little plastic baby dolls as Kenady explained how she would play a song on the cell phone to Mom and her friend, Betty. They both listened intently to every word Ken said. I saw Betty stand from her wheelchair and chuckle at Kenady and then I heard the most beautiful sound, my mother's laughter. I will hold that sound in my heart all day today. I love you Kenady. I love you mommy! Xoxo

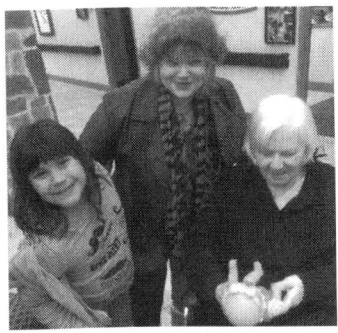

Kenady is a "natural" healer. She had so many elderly people "awake" and happy and playing with babies. She truly has a gift of love and kindness. As you can tell I am not standing up straight. Ken had run off with one of my crutches and the other one was under my left arm. See my pretty black brace on my leg? I am a real trend-setter.

NOVEMBER 30, 2014

I saw my Aunt Dot yesterday, my mom's last sibling still alive out of seven brothers and sisters. She has always been my second mom. I spent almost every summer with her and my four cousins. While visiting my Aunt we spoke about Mom. I could tell she was extremely sad and apprehensive about her visit to see her yesterday. At one point she smiled and I could see my mom in her facial expression. I had never noticed the resemblance before. It was uncanny. I told Aunt Dot this and she smiled and looked tearful at the same time. She said that once Mom was gone she would have no one left in her nucleus family. I asked her if she could be my mom too like she was every summer. She laughed her special nervous little giggle and said, "I thought I already was!" Family is so important. I don't know why we have to get older to realize this, but that is how it was for me. If I had one wish, just one, I would ask that we could have a revelation for the gifts we can receive from our elder generation and not think of them as cast aways. No matter where we hide them or ignore them, we will still get old ourselves one day. Maybe that is not a bad thing as long as someone loves you, like family. I love you, Aunt Dot. xoxo

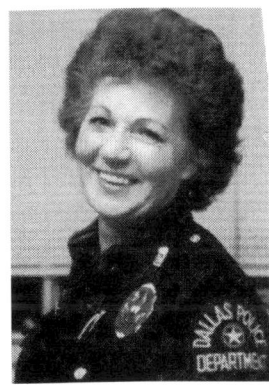

December 2, 2014

Tomorrow is my mom's 80th birthday. I am so glad she was born. If not for December 3rd, 80 years ago, the world would have missed out on an awesome police woman trail-blazing the way for other women to come forth during the fifties. She was one of those women who proved not only could a woman be a career woman, but also a mother and a wife, too. Many friends would have missed out on having a fun loving friend, who was always there for them. A young man the age of 20 would have missed out on having the love of his life marry him and have a child with him. A grand daughter and great grandchildren would have missed many hours of admiration and love from her. Many neighbors would have lost the chance to come in contact with someone who brought them pears from her own pear trees, or remembered every child's birthday on the block. A stepdaughter would have missed out on having direction in her teenage years. A Jewish man would have missed out on 26 years of being married to his soul mate. A daughter would have missed out on coming home to a dinner every afternoon waiting in the oven for her and her dad. I could go on and on. My mother is, and was, no ordinary woman. She has more life in her years than most five people have in one life. She traveled the world after she retired. She painted houses for her church. She gave and gave and never told a soul. She lived a very modest life. Although, her "mind" is fading away and much of her "true essence" is gone, it does not take away from who she is and was. I am so blessed to have had Rosemary Dedman Katzen as my mother. In my eyes you will always be alive, and well and perfect and beautiful. Happy Birthday tomorrow, Mommy! xoxo I love you forever and ever.

Lisa Churchill Miele - One of mom's dearest friends and neighbors from years ago. They have never forgotten her and come from San Antonio to visit.

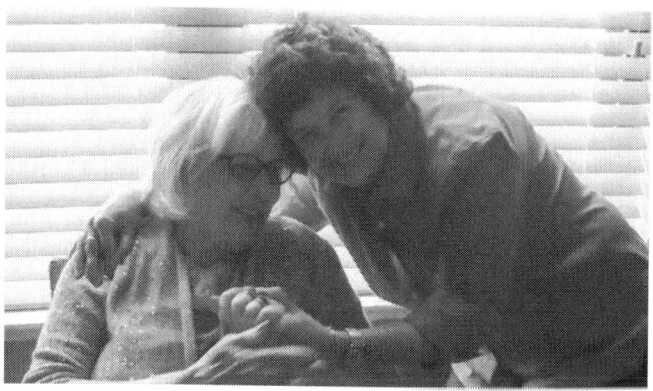

DECEMBER 4, 2014

There were about eight of us who visited Mom late afternoon on her birthday. We took a bunch of purple balloons and a huge cookie birthday cake. We tied the balloons to her wheelchair. She lay in the bed most of the time we were there. I think we over stimulated her; at times she looked like a deer in the headlights. I decided to lean over her and put my face right next to hers, kissed her and rubbed her forehead. I said, "It is ok Momma, it's Mary, and I love you." She looked at me as if to focus. She said,

"Hi darlin', I love you too." I told her how beautiful I thought she was and she held my hand tightly for a few minutes. I am so glad I was able to kiss her today and tell her I love her. I am sure Alzheimer's did not obstruct our love, not those few minutes we connected. Thank you God for those minutes. Thank you my sweet daughter for waiting on me today. I appreciate and love you. xoxoox

DECEMBER 6, 2014

Thanks for all the wonderful things posted, said, and messaged to me about the post on my mom's birthday. Sometimes I worry that I am redundant when I write. I write from my heart and from my deepest feelings. It is an out for me and I hope that it helps anyone, someone, whenever I share about anything. I am such a firm believer in love and how it heals. I have learned to pick my battles in the last few years. Life is so much easier being a lover and not a fighter! Don't get me wrong; this girl still has some fight in her when needed.

Without love, I am nothing. If I had such faith that I could move mountains, but didn't love others, I would be nothing. -1 Corinthians 13:2

DECEMBER 10, 2014

Yay me! I signed up today. I got so excited seeing the pool, I almost "accidentally" fell in. I could feel myself swimming. Gone are the days of swimming a mile in 33 minutes but that does not mean I can't get in there and still swim my a** off. I got my swim bag out of the back of the trunk of my car. I was afraid when opening it I would find spiders and cobwebs and all sorts of things, but it was all there still waiting on me. God, I can't believe I ever stopped doing something I loved so much. I thoroughly believe I just stopped living for a while because of my mother's illness. I got so focused on her care that I forgot about my own. This is not what she would want, in fact, she would be furious. Every time I swim, Mom, I will do it for you, because you can't. xoxox

DECEMBER 13, 2014

Saw my orthopedic surgeon today for a follow up on my knee and another x-ray. Today he was saying there could be a crack. I am playing truth or dare with this knee. It is either cracked or in such horrible shape they can't tell which. I am able to walk on it now, so until I can get it replaced I can deal with the pain. I am woman, hear me roar! Then I went to visit my sweet momma. She looked right at me and then looked away. She did not know me today from anyone up there. They fed her a cheeseburger and she did not eat one bite. I gave her a piece of chocolate and she did not even care. I did get a smile out of her though. I said, "Momma, I will always sneak chocolate into you, no matter what!" I rubbed her soft skin and pretended she knew me and we were having lunch together. As an only child I learned how to play "make believe." It really comes in handy these days. xoxox Lord, I am trying to find some joy in each day you give me with Mom.

DECEMBER 15, 2014

Wow, the holidays can do a number on you, can't they? I hear a Christmas carol that I have sung since I was a child and it brings all sorts of memories back. I feel so happy and then melancholy and then tearful and then sad and happy again. I am on a merry-go-round of emotions. My ruminating mind never stops. The same questions go through my mind; Will this be the last Christmas I have my mom? What should I do for her to make it a good Christmas? Alzheimer's patients don't know when tomorrow is, much less Christmas. We are down to one or two words out of her mouth with each visit, and most are mumblings and not easily understood. I feel her frustration. At times she just stops speaking all together and looks lost. I would like to know where she is. Is she in a deep dream like state? Is she trapped in her body like a butterfly trapped in a jar? These are the things I wish my analytical mind would let go of. We can guess what the brain is doing while being eaten up by this ever hungry monster disease, but "guessing" is the key word. I don't think we are afraid enough of Alzheimer's because no one can tell us how bad it is, the sufferers are unable to tell us! God, help us, if they could. I bet we would put all sorts of money into a cure. My prayer is that my mother knows nothing and she dreams her dreams, and she never has nightmares about what her life is really like. Let's all pray together for a cure. xoxoxo My memories of Christmas always include my momma, and that is a good thing.

DECEMBER 17, 2014

I got the call on the way out the door
The only words I really heard were
She is slipping away, more and more...
I was saddened, devastated drawn to my knees
God, I asked- How many more times, do I have to go through this?
Answer me please!

DECEMBER 18, 2014

When my cell phone rings, my whole body tenses up. How bad will the news be today? The calls are coming more frequent now. I have enough knowledge to know the last stage of Alzheimer's goes quickly. Each "dip" is preceded quickly by another. Last week she ate slowly, this week she is not eating on her own. Two weeks ago, she was walking, this week she is not. It would be easy to crawl into my self-pity and ask God, "How much more do you expect of me, of Mindy? How much more hurt do WE have to experience? How do you watch someone you love lose everything?" No pill, no exercise, no treatment, just the constant wait and watch as your loved one melts and fades away into nothingness. With all my will and all my might I have finally admitted to myself I am losing her to the disease. It has won and I have lost...her. It is only a matter of time now. I have never felt so helpless in my entire life. A daughter wants to pull with all her might against the inevitable of losing her beautiful mother. So, I am letting go of the ropes little by little but I am not giving her to the disease. I am lovingly handing her to God. One day at a time, Momma. I am trying to let go.

DECEMBER 22, 2014

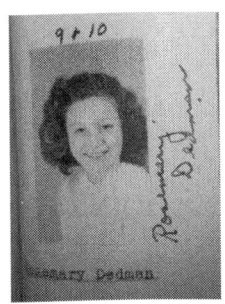

I was given a wonderful gift on Sunday. I was able to visit with my cousin, my Aunt Dot and other family members. I gave all of Mom's scarves she has worn over the years to my dear cousin, Barbara. She will try and make some kind of quilt with them. I also have the dress my mother wore when she had her retirement party after 32 years with the DPD. I am so excited to have this quilt to pass on to later generations. The thing I will cherish the most is the Annual my mother and Aunt shared. It is dated 1948-1949. My mother was so popular she was almost on every page of the annual. Of course, my mom never shared this with me. She never bragged on herself about anything! I am guessing she was about 14 years old. She was in basketball, volleyball, and a runner up for Halloween Queen Candidate. Right beside her name it states, "The twinkle in her eye spells fun." Thank you, Aunt Dot for the most awesome Christmas present. More knowledge about my mom and more information for my book, The Fading Image. xoxoxo

My Aunt Nettie, My mom, (Rose) and my Aunt Dot all on front row.

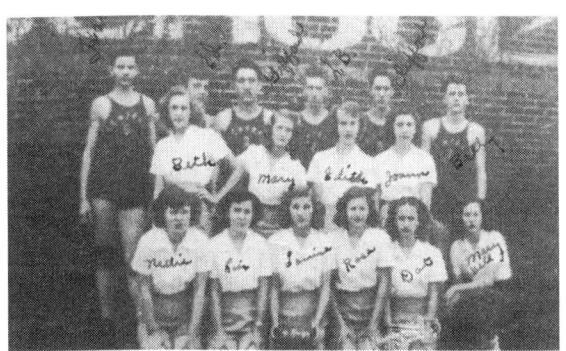

DECEMBER 23, 2014

My Mom sat pretty much motionless in her wheelchair today. Her eyes closed and merely a few whispers spoken, I began to watch her. Her hands began to move lovingly as if touching someone's face. She had a serious yet gentle look; all at once she made the motion of kissing someone. There was a moment of peace upon her beautiful face. A dream? A visit? It was a Christmas gift for me. Have sweet dreams, Momma! <3

FEBRUARY 19, 2015

My doctor recommended I stopped stressing...

My daughter (my liege) told me to get the hell out of town

My addictive self said to go gambling if I went out of town.

My loving earthly father said get your butt up here and visit me. So, in my dad's town there is a casino. I can get loved, told how awesome I am, and be a little girl. So, am I going? You bet your Goulash I am. Thanks Mindy for being my bossy girl. I love you. Xoxoxo

FEBRUARY 25, 2015

Let's pretend it is Thursday, since I will be gone tomorrow. I found about ten pictures today at Mom's. Just when I think I am going to forget how beautiful and vibrant she once was, I find a picture that reminds me of how she really is, albeit she has Alzheimer's. I don't know what year this was taken. Mindy or Jane may know. xoxo

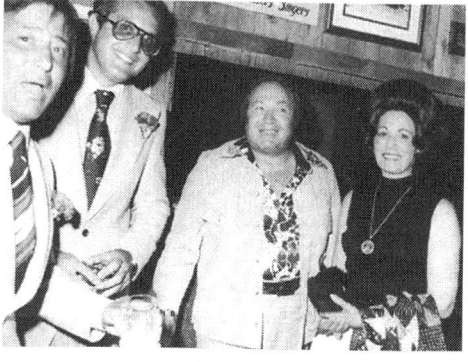

FEBRUARY 26, 2015

In my heart I believe Alzheimer's gradually takes a person's image away. They fade away slowly, and that is why I named this book "Fading Image." I found many pictures of my mom today at her house. When I do this it reminds me of whom she truly is. What a remarkable woman. Pictures are such a treasure. I felt the need to write this. I hope you enjoy it and can feel what I am saying. xoxo

I felt your true spirit today in your pictures
A picture is worth a thousand words
A photo is an image of allusion
A reminder your eyes can gaze upon
To destroy present confusion
Every time I see you it is harder to remember
When we last spoke, laughed together
 even argued...memories fading away;
But your soul still flaming inside like a burning ember
I want to take this photo of you and place upon my heartache
 and you will awaken from Alzheimer's deep sleep
Unaware of how long you have been gone or what has taken place
Reality is my enemy, almost as much as your disease
Memories of you are my saving grace
Photographs bring such pleasure
You are fading away, they never will.
Photos of you, Mom, a true treasure.

FEBRUARY 28, 2015

It had been many days since I had seen my mom, due to being out of town and the increment weather. The guilt was eating my lunch and I was missing her, although "she" is not really there. Of course, she does not know me and of course she is still digressing. Her voice is still the same, a little quieter and only disjointed sentences. If I close my eyes I can still hear my mother's voice, as if nothing has changed. It will take me at least 24 hours to get over seeing her and grieving over her again. I can understand why some family members go see their loved ones less and less. The pain is excruciating, but sometimes not seeing her is even worse.

MARCH 2, 2015

I sit here almost numb at the moment, yet it is like a tornado swarming around me. I am in the middle of it. I feel as though at any moment I will be sucked inside and thrown far, far away. *Maybe that would be a blessing*, I think to myself. I just received a call, thirty minutes ago, that my mom has fallen at her facility. They did an x-ray and she has broken her hip. An Alzheimer's patient in Hospice care now has a broken hip and is on her way to the emergency room, to get treatment for healing. It sounds like an oxymoron. Please pray for my mother, our family and extended family. They say sometimes the valley deepens before you see the sunlight. I have been praying for some sunshine. xoxox

MARCH 3, 2015

When I came on here to do an update I was shocked at all the replies. I felt like Sally Field in her Oscar nomination win years ago when she stated, "Wow, you do like me!" Mom was in surgery for about two hours. They did a partial hip replacement and she is now in recovery. Upon leaving the hospital, she will be in a skilled nursing home for about thirty days, and then moved to a nursing home and out of memory care. I guess she is now on her way to the last house on the block, so to speak. If any of you are aware of a caring, and good quality nursing home facility please message me. We need something in the Garland area so she will be close to us. Hospice is helping us look also. We have about thirty days to find another facility. God bless Hospice and God bless the doctors and nurses at Presby. Oh, and God bless all the awesome people who truly care on Facebook. <smoochies>

I thank the Lord for those friends who can pray for me when I can't even find these words for myself. xoxoxo

Jesus said, the greatest of these is LOVE...

MARCH 4, 2015

The outpouring of suggestions and love for my mom has been overwhelming. She had a pretty tough time last night with some heart issues but is stable today. Due to all the suggestions on Facebook, I have contacted different home based care places. Mindy and I will be looking at these homes tomorrow that care for Alzheimer's patients. I never knew these places existed. There is so much out there that caregivers and families of those who need care do not know about. This is a shame. I continue to meet the most awesome and caring individuals during this journey with my mom. Thank you Trish for all your help today. Thank you again to those at Hospice and thank you to everyone on Facebook who sends me love in your comments and texts. I am so truly blessed. I want to be a blessing to you, too. Just let me. xoxoxo

MARCH 5, 2015

Today, Mindy and I are on our quest to find Mom a new residence. I wish we had known about these homes a year or so ago. Of course we would all like to keep our parents with us at home as long as we can, but some illnesses do not afford us that luxury. Parents out there please sit down with your adult children and tell them your wishes. We, as your children, are not mind readers. We let our love for you get in the way. We think with our hearts and not with our brains. Of course it is a sad and tough issue to discuss, but death and dying is a natural part of our lives. Since we, as parents, do love our children and we, as adult children, do adore our parents, please take time to speak with a parent or child about their wishes, their financial plans, and their funeral wishes. It is a part of loving them and making sure everyone is on the same page. I use to tell my parents, "I don't want to talk about it." I would tell anyone today, talk about it. Discuss it until you have it down by memory. When we are losing you, we can barely function much less try and decide what your wishes were. My mother had a Will, a Directive, prenuptial agreement, a Power of Attorney and hand written letters. I think she had every legal document available. Thank you, Mom!!! xoxo You don't know how many times this has helped me when someone asked me what we needed to do. I was able to answer without wondering if I was doing what my mom wanted.

MARCH 5, 2015
Well, I just got off the phone with the Director over the Memory Care Unit where Mom was for 2 1/2 years. We cried, we laughed and we decided we would definitely keep in touch. It seems no matter where my mother goes in her life she always touches the people she comes in contact with. I mainly knew my mom as my mom. I am learning all about her as a friend to others, as a neighbor, and just a genuinely nice, engaging person. It is so strange to get to know who she was aside from being "Mom." This journey she and I have traveled has been one of acceptance for me. Most of my life I feared getting older, and feared death above all else. I no longer have this horrific fear of old age. I have seen my mom travel that path with grace and dignity through this horrible disease. I still fear death, but am coming to an understanding of it. My mom still teaches me lessons every day.

Thank you, Rebecca, for loving my mom and for caring for her, that means so much. xoxoxo

That's how it will be when our bodies are raised to life. "These bodies will die, but the bodies that are raised will live forever. These ugly and weak bodies will become beautiful and strong. As surely as there are physical bodies, there are spiritual bodies. And our physical bodies will be changed into spiritual bodies." 1 Corinthians 15: 42-44

MARCH 6, 2015
I dislike "goodbyes." Even as a child they gave me such an empty feeling in my gut. If I saw a neighbor packing up and moving from our block I felt such loss inside. It was

like a part of me was going to be missing. Funny how everyone you meet makes up whom you are. Everyone I have met in my life has taught me something. I will miss so many of my mom's old friends at her prior residence. Those she laughed with, played games with and even danced and sang with. I will miss those caregivers and staff members who have a job that is low paying, hard work, but rewarding in many ways to them and to family members. I will always miss Diamond yelling, "Rosie!" I will miss Betty and her smile, and all the sweet, lovely people who find such joy in just a little bit of human kindness. There are also those special people who I believe God has chosen to be in the caregiving field. They have a calling for this type of work. You can see it in the way they are when they are with Alzheimer's patients. They have the patience of Job. Their ministry is in their profession. Although I am thankful for Mom's new "home" and the new friends she will make today, I am still feeling that same feeling I felt as a child. Someone is moving away from my life and it is truly sad. When I go there today to gather my mother's belongings, it will be hard to say goodbye without getting to say goodbye to all these wonderful people I have grown to love who only know me on the day I come. They will not feel the loss I will be feeling, and for that, I am grateful. xoxo

MARCH 6, 2015

On Tuesday I asked a friend how much more God wants my family to go through. How much more does my mother have to suffer? I was in one of my "poor me" modes. Her answer was, until God is ready. Each day God shows me more of His love through others. I always knew there were loving people in this world. I have become more hardened due to things going on in the world; the atrocities, the killings, our own government. At times I have lost faith in the goodness of certain entities. But, those are just things that really have nothing to do with the broad brush of human kindness. Today, my mother was sent to her new facility without her dentures. The follow up papers read, "Patient will need to eat pureed food." It also stated she was not eating. Gee, I wonder why? Of course I was livid. My anger usually comes from fear or from exasperation of neglect of any kind. *What do I do*, I ask myself. The only thing I could think of was to call Hospice. I spoke with Amanda. These angels seem to never take a break. She answers even when she should be off work. I tell her the situation and she tells me she will go to the hospital room and check for me. Maybe, just maybe, they will still be there. A few minutes later I get a text, "I have them." I felt the anguish leave me. My mom does not eat much these days, can't chew well and can hardly swallow. But, I could not imagine her having to eat pureed food, plus another loss of her dignity, no dentures. Amanda took these aged, white pearlies to my mom's new residence. I asked her why she would make such a long trip to do this for us on such short notice. Her answer, "I thought about what I would want for my own mother in the same situation." God is still teaching me all about love, and I thought I knew everything already. Silly, silly me. xoxoxo

MARCH 7, 2015

I think God opened up the skies and dropped angels down in human form and decided they would be called members of Hospice. I know each one by name who has stepped into my mother's descending process. Those names are etched upon my heart forever. I think Alzheimer's is winning now. My mother is weary and exhausted by it. She is not doing well and rarely opens her eyes now. My mother has a directive that says, no this, no that, etc. I thought I could be strong and go by her wishes to the letter. The mind listens to her wishes but my heart is breaking at her requests. Just the thought of her being gone, imagine the reality of it. I was given a paper that says, "Signs and symptoms of approaching death," today I am unable to read it past the first paragraph. Maybe tomorrow. I will go by her wishes even though it makes me want to pull my heart out of my chest so I no longer feel this terrible pain. Love is a powerful thing, no wonder we want to never let go of those who have shown us so much. I love you Momma, I will see you tomorrow. It will be ok. I promise. xoxoxo Thanks, Katrina DeAnn Montenegro.

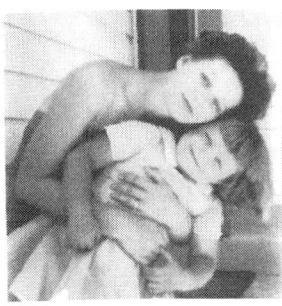

Mommy, mother, friend....
The bond transcends.
Roles may be reversed
But, the love never ends.
Not ever...

MARCH 8, 2015

Jane, Mindy and I spent time with Mom today. Thank you Debby, another angel. I really cannot even express the love I am getting from everyone. I feel like sometimes people are probably sick of my sad posts. If you get anything from my posts please see past my sadness and just relish in all the love coming from others to me, someone hurting. You guys are the best medicine I am getting right now. I pray for everyone who is walking through this with me. I even told my mom about all of you today. They say she can hear me. You are bringing joy to her too. Thank you. You are true blessings to my whole family; they are all reading my posts.

If I can be only half the woman she was and is, then I am everything I could ever hope to be. xoxoox

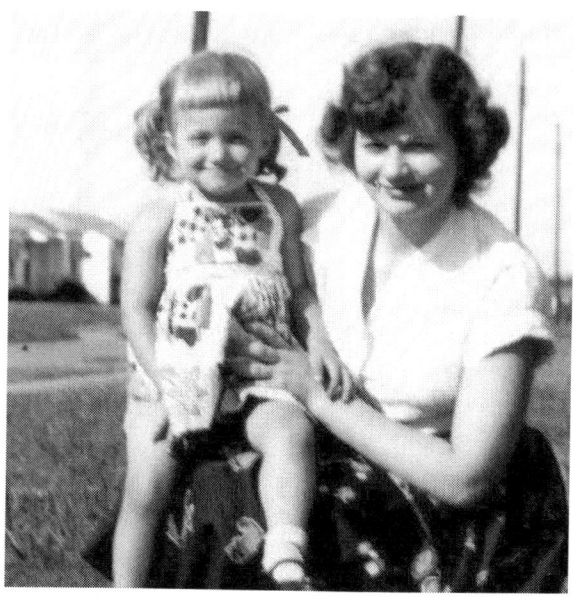

MARCH 10, 2015

These last days
And the angels came, sat by the bed
With a cool cloth soothed her head.
Touching her body as though it was sacred
As she laid there, any pain, God would forbid.
I sit beside her with all my regrets
My tears falling upon her chest.
I imagine her waking and giving me a kiss
But her lifeless body, laying here, is all I get.
Regrets, remorse, gut wrenching pain
Is this really what God ordained?
To consecrate such sadness to those left behind
At once I feel a touch upon my hand
I turn my face and there an angel stands
She explains to me that God would not let me weep
But find joy in my mother's final sleep

Don't listen to all those other lies
You can conjure up in your mind
Listen instead to your heart
The words of your loving God.
Let us (Hospice) take care of your mom.
Thank you God for your earthly angels...

MARCH 10, 2015

Today was an awesome day in many ways. I gathered up white roses I had and a beautifully scented Hyacinth I had grown. They smell Heavenly. I also took some of Mom's favorite color of fingernail polish with me. When I got there she was having more problems breathing but seemed without stress. I took off her old polish, filed her nails and painted them a beautiful shade of red. I then moved down to her feet. At eighty years old her feet look like they belong to a 30 year old. Not one crooked piggy in the group. I then took the rose petals and sprinkled them all over her. As I was doing all these things, I was telling her what I was doing. "Mom, I am covering you with rose petals." "Mom, I am painting your toe nails red." "Mom, I am painting your fingernails red." "Mom, I sprayed perfume on you, you smell so good!" I then got into the bed with her, being very careful of her hip, and put my arm across her ever-thinner chest and hugged her like I did as a child. I did not cry. I was quiet. At that moment I heard her make a deep groan. I got up slowly and before I left I put the Hyacinth to her nose. I said, "Smell this Momma, it smells like you always smelled to me...beautiful." she let out another deep groan. Was she responding to me? I would like to think so. When I am with her, I am ok with her going. When I am away from her I want her to stay, so I may see her again. I told her I would see her tomorrow, but if she had to go to please come see me in my dreams. xoxox

MARCH 11, 2015

This will be the last entry about my beautiful mother's disease of Alzheimer's and how she and I fought back against it as much as we could. My mom has passed. I think mom was just waiting for me to polish her nails and cover her with roses. I guess now I can see her in my dreams and now she will be well. I always wanted that and she did too. Dance, Mommy, dance. We both appreciate all the love on here and now she too can read all the beautiful things that were said about her. Please help me with my fight against this horrible disease.

MARCH 12, 2015

Yesterday, as I was painting her nails and had placed all the white rose buds all over her body, I played the song by Plumb, "Lord, I Am Ready Now." She again let out this deep groan. Does anyone know how to put that song on my Facebook page? She was so beautiful when Jesus came to get her. I can just see her now being lifted from her bed with the roses falling off of her. God, thank you for giving me the love of a mother. Rest in peace, Mommy.

Mindy and I were together today
We were crying over you
We found soiled clothes of yours
They needed to be washed
We threw them out the window
As we drove down the street
I cry over you in waves
Mindy is like you so much
But, guess she is just like me, too
I look at your pictures now trying to find the "right" one
They are all beautiful, just like you
The kids ask about you and most likely always will
Dad misses you too, God, the men sure love you.
You were a man magnet, mom. Let's face it.
I hope you liked the roses yesterday
I think I got your feet, Mindy sure did not!
She got Evelyn's, HA HA
OK, I know you are busy and Heaven is awesome for sure
I feel better knowing you are out of those damn wrinkly clothes
You can put on your own makeup, brush your own teeth, your OWN teeth
Save me a place in line, will you? I love you

MARCH 12, 2015

Again, let me reiterate. I cannot believe the love I am receiving from everyone. At times I feel like I am sitting on a barrel full of hot coals. Other times I keep thinking I need to do something for Mom. It has been years that I have not needed to do something for her, to protect her in some way. I feel lost. As soon as the dust settles I intend to find some way to help caregivers. My book is only my beginning to help those suffering as I was. The times I feel the most "safe" are when I read your love. God help me to be ok with just being a "being," and not doing all the time.

MARCH 12, 2015

I call Mindy first thing this morning and the first thing she said was, "I smelled Nanny last night; that old grandma perfume smell." I started laughing.

I explained I put a new fresh smelling perfume on her the last day I was with Mom. Mindy was like, "No, it was her old perfume." I said, "Damn, she came to see you AGAIN?" Mom died at 6:00am on Monday. Mindy woke up, no alarm, right out of bed at 6:00am. Me, I was sawing logs. I did not smell any perfume last night either. I told Mindy, there you guys go again, with that special bond you have. Mindy laughed and said, "Well, this time you can have these "visits." I don't want that kind of stuff" I started kidding her and said, "Well, you should not have bonded with her so much in the real world." I will take the old grandma perfume, the waking up and even a visit or two. But, you know what, it will probably be Mindy getting the visits. I thoroughly understand. I am CRAZY about my grandbabies too. Probably when I am gone I will come see them instead of Mindy. There is just that special thing about your grandbaby. Sorry, Mindy, you better just get used to it. Oh, tell Mom, "Hi", next time she comes by. xoxoox

MARCH 12, 2015

Stages of my grief

At this point, I cannot stand to be asked a question, any question. When I am it is like someone is asking me the question from a room at the other end of a building. I hear the words but I am thinking to myself, *please stop talking; I have to listen for my mother.* I want to go places but I can't seem to get ready to do it. The days are long, and yet I can't believe it was just yesterday she passed. It seems like it was over a week ago. The only time I feel less pain is when I am with Mindy, Bradyn or Kenady, but primarily Mindy. I feel safe talking to my family, other police officers and really close friends. But, the pain only subsides when I am with Mindy. She is the Band-Aid on my loss right now. I am so glad my dad is coming into town. I will be so glad to see family and friends and comrades of Mom. I am just hurting now and needed to write about it. I am so glad she is free. Mom, don't be mad at me because I am missing you. I know you are much better off. I just realize now that even though you were not yourself, I still had a mom. I miss you.

To mom...I KNOW you can hear me.

Mom…I know you are mad
You said, no flowers, no Urn,
Just Tupperware.
Don't spend a penny more than what I already paid
Mom, that was fifteen years ago, times have changed!
I will put Mindy in charge of funeral plans
She can say no, and you can't.
You're too sensitive!
She sure fooled you.
Guess what, when it comes to you
She is sensitive too!
We even rented a room at Holiday Inn
We ordered some food too
It's not our fault so many loved you
Are you gonna be mad at me, oh wow!
That is not Heavenly or humane.
Remember where you are now?
You have to set an example for others you know
We just could not place you in a Tupperware bowl.
I promise I will recycle your clothes, sell your chair for a dollar
Take care of all your birds outside, water all your flowers
I bought my dress on sale that I will be wearing Sunday
Does that make you feel more at ease?
Better talk to Mindy, she did not get hers on sale. heeheehee
See, I AM the one you should have really liked the best. See, see!
I guess I will keep writing you till I don't think you can hear me anymore. xoxo

MARCH 13, 2015

I will begin to post pictures of Mom's friends on Facebook. These are some of her favorite policewomen she worked with, Jean, Mary, Patsy and Becky. She loved these women as friends and as co-workers. xoxo

Co-workers

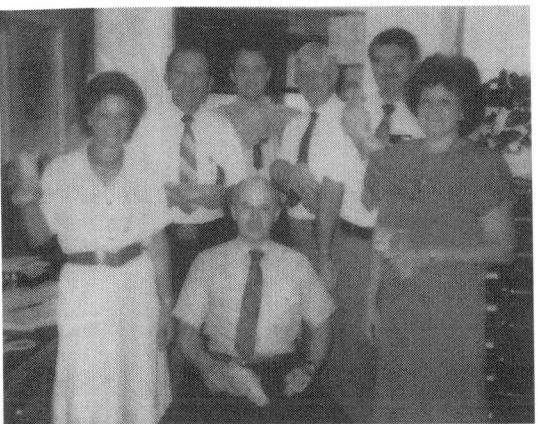

All five sisters

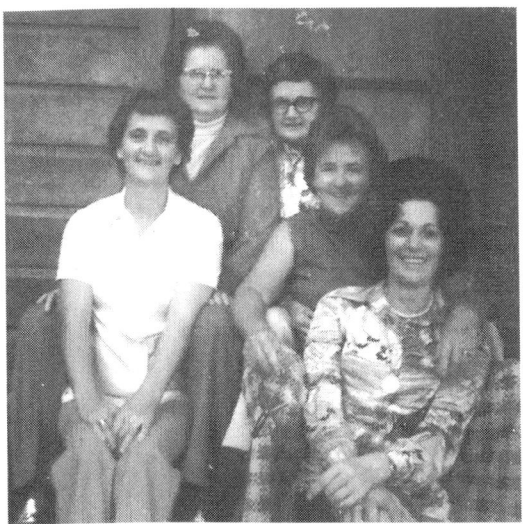

MARCH 13, 2015

My sweet Mindy is here and we are going through pictures. My mom's neighbor, David Jayakaran, who lived across the street from her, is officiating the celebration of her life. She adored him. He visited her many times and prayed with her often. They were also instrumental in helping me to get guardianship of my mother. There are so many people I have to thank for helping me in our long and arduous journey her last few years. We not only fought the battle of Alzheimer's, but personal battles as well. This happens many times to the elderly and those who have decreased mental capabilities. If you have an elderly parent, please stay close to them and beware of monsters out there, they do exist. Those you least expect, even banks can sometimes be the worst predators. There is money that can be gained by talking an elderly person into putting their money in certain funds. This change can sometimes not be an earning for them but for the person at the bank making the change. The elderly are very susceptible to this abuse and then you add the disease of Alzheimer's and you have a perfect combination for financial misuse. We were dealing with issues from many areas in her life that (before Alzheimer's) she had total control over, now she had none.

My mother was safe the last three years of her life. She was back in the arms of her beloved family. I cannot even begin to thank those who were so instrumental in helping us help her. There is a list of them beginning with caregivers, police officers, neighbors, attorney's, court investigators, APS, friends and the list goes on. I cherished every day that I had with my mom thanks to all of you. Blessings. xoxoox

MARCH 14, 2015

I just got a call from the DPD. There will be an honor guard tomorrow folding and refolding a flag and then given to me. This I knew about. Taps will be played after. I also found out a Texas flag will be flown over the capital for a few days and then taken down, folded and sent to me. I am overwhelmed. It is like I told David who is officiating the ceremony. I knew my mom as my mommy. I have only recently, in the last few years come to know her as the professional woman she was. In 2012 when we first placed her in Memory Care, we gave her that surprise birthday party. The next day we were with her putting all her cards away. She looked at Mindy and I and asked, "Who had a birthday?" I knelt down and looked at her and said it was her birthday. I began to tell her what a wonderful woman she was, how she had changed the world for other women in her field. How a skinny farm girl had left Arkansas and made it to Dallas to become one of the first police officers. She got a tear in her eye, my mother rarely cried, she looked at me and said, "I was just doing my job, Mary" That was my mother. I will be with you tomorrow, Momma. xoxox

MARCH 14, 2015

Please forgive this announcement on Facebook but I can't call all family members. Please understand I am an only child, Mindy is an only granddaughter. We are planning this in a matter of days. The service, the reception, pictures, music, contacts and moving her from memory care to a group home and then to a funeral parlor in a matter of one week. If I cannot meet with family members coming into town tonight or first thing in the morning, please do not feel like I am unkind or unloving or ungrateful.

These are the reasons we planned things at Holiday Inn, rooms and reception. Mindy and I will give you our full attention tomorrow and we plan to spend as much time as humanly possible with everyone celebrating Mom's life after the services and at the reception. I am so grateful for anyone that is attending; it is just taking every second we have to finish everything. Love, Mary and Mindy Michelle Stevens

MARCH 14, 2015

Well I am off to bed. Tomorrow will be a great day for me. I can put my mother to rest and start the healing process. I will finish my book with the help of my publisher. I intend to do what I can for other caregivers out there and to also help fight the good fight against Alzheimer's disease. If you have a loved one who is a caregiver or if you, yourself are one, please contact me. If you have a loved one who suffers with AD, please contact me. Just because the journey with my beloved mother has ended does not mean my story is over. If you need help in finding a safe place for a loved one, give me a call or write me. I am here for all those out there who need help. I will carry on the memory of my beautiful mother who could have lived years longer had she not fought against a relentless foe. We will win one day against this disease. Caregivers do need our help; let's not forget them. Elder abuse does happen. Love and care for one another. Regrets are non-refundable. Love, M xoxoxo

MARCH 16, 2015

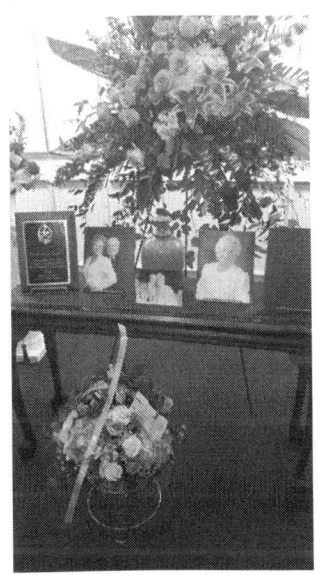

I was blessed beyond means today. I gave my mother to Jesus and walked away. I am working now on letting her go. That gap, emptiness, and hollowness will take time to fill itself up. All I can say is that I was blessed to the further side of reality by what happened to me today. I was reintroduced to old family members from Arkansas that I had never even met before. I come from a huge family and yet I know very few of them, and have seen very few of them since I was a baby. I saw them today and I adored them. My mother's ex-husband (my dad), attended her funeral and he saw her old comrades who remembered him. Can you believe that? I saw some of her old boyfriends. They told me while they were dating her, if I called, she would drop everything to call me back. I came first. I met those that loved her, adored her and thought she dripped with integrity, love and loyalty. A neighbor officiated her cele-

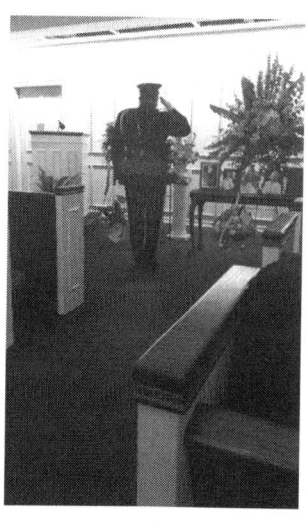

bration and cried while doing so. I listened to caregivers, friends, police officers and nurses talk about her sense of fairness and her sense of humor. I fell in love with my mother all over again today. When the honor guards folded her flag I was first, proud of my country, second, proud of the force and thirdly, proud of my mother who served it so well. As they played taps and refolded the flag we all cried. When the guard got down on his knees, handed me the flag and thanked my mom for her service, I felt such an honor just to have known her much less be her daughter. I cannot thank the police force enough for what they gave to me today. The love I received from my friends and family and the love I have received from Facebook is overwhelming. I am hurting, that is for sure, I am so blessed and so thankful to be alive and to be so loved by so many. Thank you. I am humbled. Xoxoxo

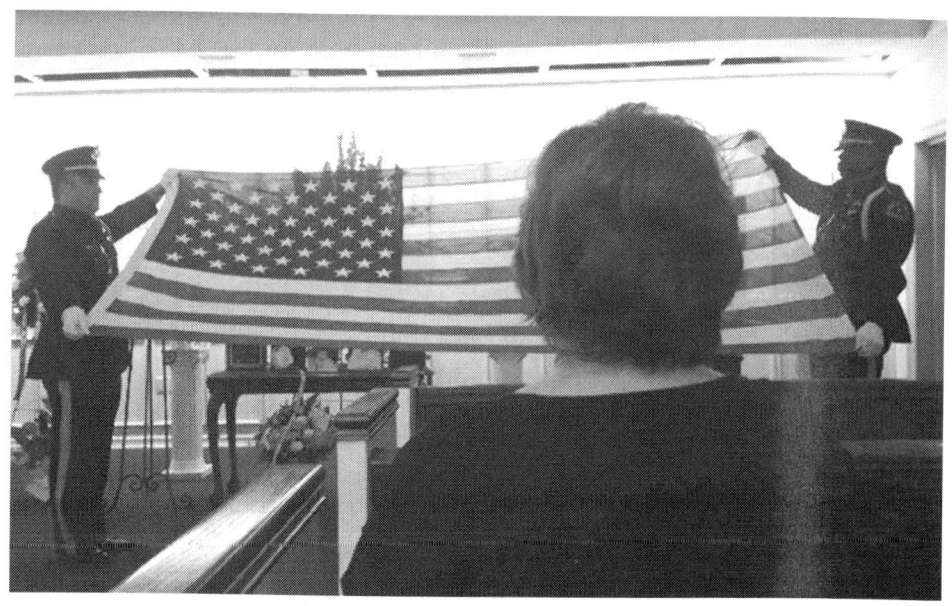

My rock

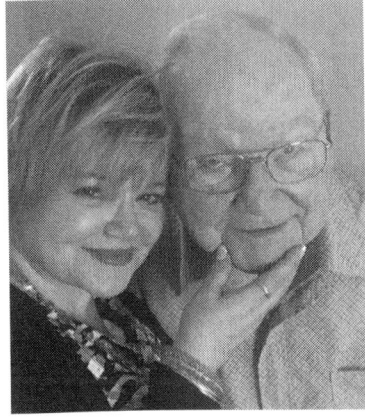

Me and my dad, Ray Birdwell

MARCH 16, 2015

Sweet Karen to the rescue today. Xxox

Me and Karen Babb

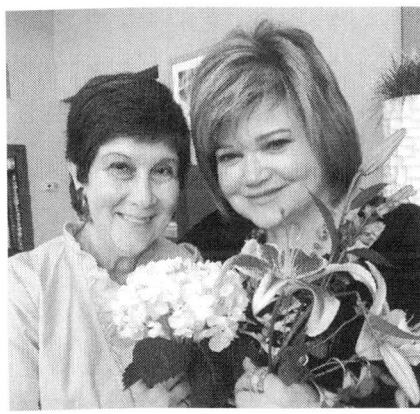

MARCH 17, 2015

Grief is horrible. You think you just made it over a hill and then you look up and there is a mountain in front of you to climb. I do not know how "long time" spouses manage after losing their life partners. I have such a new understanding of so many things. I will never negate another's feelings of loss, or tell them it is time to move on. I hope I have never done that. I am so raw and I am sure I am not pleasant to be around right now. It comes and it goes. I pray for all those who are hurting right now, please have peace and know that I am praying for you and for me. xoxoxo

MARCH 17, 2015

Mindy and I will pick up Mom's remains tomorrow at noon. We have planned our own little ceremony. We had Mom's thumb prints made into charms; one for me, Jane and Mindy. I also got a teardrop and Mindy got a cross, each will contain some of Mom's cremations. This way she will always be close to us. I want to find a beautiful garden somewhere to spread her ashes and one other place she requested. We are going to carry all of her flowers from the service and place those at different spots too. Some I will save for her own garden, which I think it will be a lovely tribute to her. Each day it is like a puzzle; the heart breaks apart and you gradually put each piece back in place. I will be a better person after this journey. I will be better at helping others who grieve, better at feeling other's pain, and better at having been loved when it was needed the most.

MARCH 17, 2015

Sometimes I/we get so wrapped up in our own pain we forget others are hurting too. I got a message tonight from a dear friend who has more on her plate than a Roman at a food orgy. When I listened to her hurts I felt the majority of mine disappear. I had such empathy for her. We all have our own laundry, our own tears and our own fears. Yes, I have lost my mom, yes, I am in pain, but when I reached out to another tonight, my pain lifted and I actually felt relief. Giving is so healing.

"While we have opportunity, let us do good to all people." -Galatians 5:10

MARCH 18, 2015
Mom's shadow box at Memory Care unit.

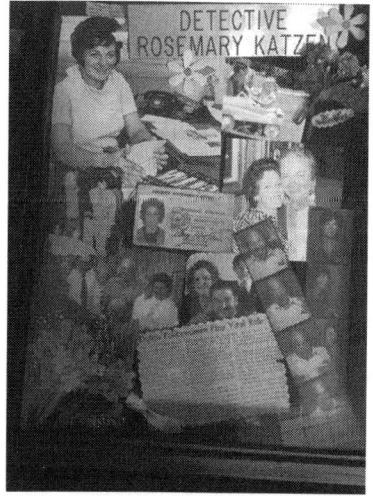

MARCH 18, 2015

Well, Mindy and I said our final "goodbye" to Mom today. I have my teardrop charm with some of her ashes and Mindy has her cross charm. I honestly feel as if a weight has been lifted off me and she has flown away free. Each time Mindy and I take care of "one more thing," it helps us to let go more and more. We are trying to respect all of her final wishes. We visited Murray's, gravesite today and placed some flowers from her funeral there. Now, we feel we can visit the two of them at one time. It is all a process. I will let my body be in motion to proceed to finish a few last things, tie up some lose ends and make Rosemary's Garden a beauty to behold. Her ashes will become some of the newest blooms in her garden. Bye, Momma. I am so glad you are finally free. Dance all you want to. I am beginning to feel so happy for you. xoxo

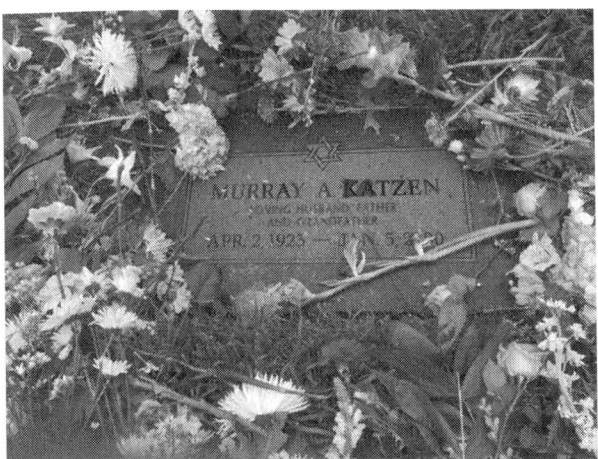

Mom and Murray together....

MARCH 19, 2015

I think it just hit me right now. I am exhausted. I was already an ADD type of person, but the last few weeks I think I have been ADD on Espresso. I make so many spelling mistakes, date mistakes, day mistakes; I even told everyone at Mom's funeral the wrong day she passed. I wish I had an anchor or some type of heavy weight so I could wrap it around my head and sit still somewhere. If you ask me a question please don't expect a tried and true answer for a few weeks. I don't even think I know who I am right now. Love, Sara Jane

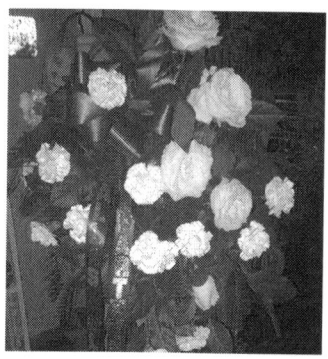

MARCH 20, 2015

I was doing pretty well today and then someone at Walmart was complaining about a police officer and I just lost it inside. It was like they stuck a knife in my heart. I have always taken up for our guys and gals in blue and always will, but this was just not the time. Came home and cried like a baby, texted a Hospice angel, and probably woke the poor angel up. I won't do that again, but I am better now. I also took Mom's spray down from her front porch. I took a picture of it; I wish I had taken the picture before it started wilting. Oh well, it still looks pretty after so many days. I will save the flowers and use them as fertilizer in her garden. xoxo

MARCH 22, 2015

A work still in progress. Look at the sun shining right down on the first flowers I planted for her. I am still planting a little each day. Rosemary's Garden is a work in progress. I had to share the sun coming out and shining on the bed of flowers. xoxoxo

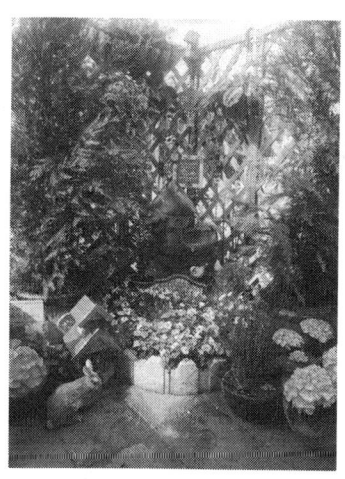

MARCH 22, 2015

I am getting sympathy cards from cousins in Arkansas. I have not seen them in years and years. The first sentence is always, I remember Aunt Rosemary as being so beautiful, so funny and on and on. Her favorite brother, Scooter's, two children wrote me. I was floored to hear from them. I wanted to contact them but did not know how, neither did Mom. After her brother died, we lost contact. Now I can contact them. If there is one lesson I have learned and would like to pass on it is this, stay in touch with your family, write often, and don't wait until you lose someone for everyone to make contact again. Family is forever. xoxo

MARCH 23, 2015

We all celebrated a friend's birthday last night. Kenady calmly says, "Mommy, did you tell GG that Nana talked to you in a dream? I sat up like a "Jack in the Box." "What, what, what?" The last sentence I said to my mom was, "Please come see me in my dreams if you leave me." Of course she was semi-conscious. I will never know if she heard me. Mindy calmly said, "Oh yeah, she came to me in a dream last night." I was about to have a coronary; I wanted to hear everything, twice! She said, Nanny looked about thirty years old, had dark hair and they talked without talking. My mom was laughing about what we did with her ashes and how Mindy had inhaled some of them. She said we did everything right. She spoke about hating her diseased body and how glad she was to be out of it. She said she was so happy now. Mindy said they laughed a lot and when she woke up she started crying over the dream. I was so happy to hear that Mom had visited Mindy. I am so happy we did everything right and that Mom was so glad to be free of her Alzheimer's. Last night in the car, I spoke to my mom. I asked her to come and see me in a dream, in a vision, anywhere and anytime. I talk to her a lot. I feel like now she understands every word I say. Those years with Alzheimer's I felt I was talking to her disease, today I feel I am talking to my momma. My grief is still so fresh but my love for her is everlasting. Don't get me wrong, I am so happy for her. I would not change one thing, except just loving her more. If that were possible. xoxoxo

MARCH 24, 2015

It is not the sad memories of losing my mom that keep me awake at night, it is the memories of her just being here, just having a mother. My mother would have given anything to keep her memory. Yet, it is the memories that cause me the most pain right now. But, I would not want those taken from me for anything. Alzheimer's does that and it does not care whom it chooses to be its victim. I pray for peace for all those victims of this horrible disease and for those caregivers dealing with the loss of those they love.

Mom, please be patient with me.

I peruse the cards, read a few,

Pack them away,

I will read them tomorrow, maybe

Just not today.

As I folded your clothes,

I experienced a whiff of you

I immediately wished

I was helping to dress you

Like I used to.

I keep thinking in my mind

I just want to hold your hand

Be with you, ONE more time.

I know this is better for all involved

I know it is, I know it is.
I know, Mom

MARCH 25, 2015

I feel the need to post this. I am not doing so to apologize to anyone. I just want the facts out there. My mom fell and broke her hip on March 2nd of this month. She was immediately transferred to the hospital. They operated next the morning doing a partial hip replacement. The night after surgery she almost died. My mother never fully regained consciousness. During this time our family moved her furniture and belongings from the Memory Unit. She was transferred to the new group home on Friday, March 7th. We moved all of her belongings to the new residence. Hospice followed. We decorated her new room, bought her new clothes and awaited her arrival on Sunday. She never awoke again, never talked again, never ate on her own again. She was unable to swallow as of Monday the 9th. She was hooked up to oxygen, given morphine and lovingly taken care of by Hospice, my daughter and myself. She passed, by the grace of God, on Wednesday morning of the 11th. On that day we went to the funeral home, made arrangements and had her celebration of life on Sunday. This all happened in a matter of eleven days. Mindy and I went exactly by my mother's wishes on everything; her DNR orders, her ashes and her funeral. If someone feels, or wants to call me in the future and make claims that I did not "let them know" about the funeral, then let me give you my sincerest apologies. I was rather busy taking care of my mom for the last few years and then the last few hours of her life.

MARCH 28, 2015

We had a prayer group meeting at Mom's house last night. David, who officiated Mom's service, led the meeting. It was a blessing to all who attended. We discussed our ideas of Heaven and the great love that God has for each of us. I could easily feel my mother's presence. I needed this meeting last night. There has always been a web of protection around me, Mindy and Mom. There were/are so many people who played such an integral part in her life from 2010 up until she passed. A few months before the incident in February of 2010 with the Silver Alert and the train incident I had already started months before to get help for her situation. After the train incident, I was determined to get guardianship. Yesterday, I emailed one of the first people that helped us in our endeavor to protect her from further harm. I wanted her to know Mom had passed. I received an email back today. She and I kept up with one another over the years. She genuinely had a great heart for those in possible harm. There were people specifically sent from God to help us along this last journey of her life. When I look back at all she/

we went through, we ended our journey with a victorious outcome. She was so blessed beyond my wildest imagination. When I awoke this morning I read the returned email. It was from an angel of many. The last sentence in the email to me was this:

"Your mother accomplished many great things in her life-most importantly children who loved and cared for her. Take care and all the best."

Me....

God continues to bless me and surround me with loving and caring people. If I did not have love from others, I truly would be nothing. xoxoo

MARCH 30, 2015

I walked tonight and the sky was beautiful. I could see the stars and the wind was lightly blowing. It was crisp and clean. I love spring. As I walked I looked up at the sky and I spoke to my mom. I feel her around me all the time. It is a light presence. I am never afraid or feel encumbered. I talk to her like she is right beside me. I am at the age I am now but she is actually younger than me, yet she is still my mother; just as wise as she always was. There is nothing between us but complete unconditional love. She is free and happy. I hope this feeling never leaves me. I have come to believe this is most likely God as an intercessor between my mom and me. I know God is not a "person" per se. But, I believe he knows what I need. Who but God would know that I NEED to believe my mom is safe, happy, free, around me, watching me and with me at all times. God is all of these and so what if he brings that message to me through my mom or for my mom...it still gets to my heart. Thank you God for helping to heal my heart a little at a time every day. xoxox

I pray for all of us who are healing from losing someone, whether it was yesterday or fifty years ago. I am still praying for all the caregivers too. Much love to you and prayers that you are granted some time alone. xoxo

APRIL 2, 2015

I feel like the baton has been passed to me. Before Mom got sick she would make these huge meals and we would get together for holidays. She made weird combinations of foods. I think it was to try and accommodate every one. Murray would always make fun of her cooking. He called it her Arkansas country cooking. He sure ate lots of it as he complained. She used paper towels instead of napkins and he went on and on about that also. I would give anything to hear them play argue with one another again. I can't decide if I want to cook or not. Mindy always does the Thanksgiving thing. When Mom got sick we just took our meals to the center or went out to eat. It just made it easier. I don't know if I will cook this holiday or maybe wait until Mother's Day. Either way, I intend to use paper towels as napkins. I just need someone to complain about me doing it. I am SURE I can talk Mindy into doing that.

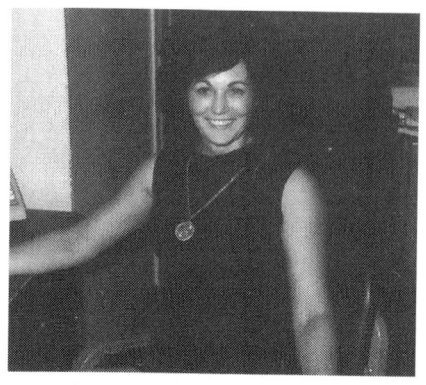

APRIL 3, 2015

After losing someone, you don't just say "goodbye" and move on. There really is no time for feeling sad. I think I am just as busy as before. I was taking care of her, and now I am taking care of her things. I have come across so many things. Mom's whole past lays inside these walls, in these boxes, her decorations, her clothes, she is still everywhere. I believe a part of me has not given up on the idea that she is still in Memory Care waiting for me to come and visit. It was a long journey for Mom and me. I think our tour of Alzheimer's was one of dignity and grace, as much as one can experience such a thing. When I look back on our goals and what we accomplished, I think we definitely made a good team. Me, Mom and Mindy. As I look and find new pictures of her, I am still taken back at her beauty, her contagious smile and the pure loveliness of her. I was/am so blessed to have had her as my mother.

APRIL 3, 2015

I picked Kenady up today and we went to have a pedicure and get our nails done. We both got "Hello Kitty" on our big toe and little polka dots on the other ones. Yep, you heard me. An eight year old and a forty plus year old. People looked at my toes and loved them. All the mature women in the place were saying, "I want that!" You know, I don't know who made up the rules that you have to be a certain age to wear this or do that, but I stopped listening to rule makers a long time ago. I don't intend to ever dress my age, look my age or especially act my age My Mom use to always tell me I worried too much about what people thought. She would be so proud of me today for getting "Hello Kitty" on my toes. Ok, I am stretching it a bit. But, she would be thrilled that I don't give a rat's behind if someone does not like it.

APRIL 5, 2015

I want to say a special thank you to my cousin, Barbara Patterson. Needless to say, the last few weeks I have not had my head screwed on straight. Most times I go to my "fear" mode when in stress. Although, I am picking door #1 more often now. The GOD door, the door of faith and no fear. My JOY runneth over, in regards to the awesome people who have been placed in my life, Barbara being one of them. Suffice it to say, I trusted and still trust her with my most valuable treasures. She and I know exactly what I am referring to. I am so blessed to have her as a member of my family and to also call my "sister" in Christ. Yesterday was one of those days I let fear grab me like a rabid dog. As soon as she called I felt myself relax, let go and gain my sense of wellness again. Friends and family are like that. They are always there for us, always loving unconditionally, and we are always blessed by them.

APRIL 7, 2015

I have my next to the last appointment tomorrow at two dentist's offices. This implant business has not been a lot of fun. I am almost a year into it now. I will not miss my wonderful flipper. I cannot wear it when I eat. I don't know how many times I have wrapped it in a disinfectant cloth and stuck it in my purse when going out to eat. It holds two teeth right next to the front teeth, and stays in there magically. I wish I could count the times I have smiled at a waiter or waitress and forgotten that I had taken it out of my mouth. I don't know who was more surprised, them or me! I can't count the amount of times I have left the house and remembered a few miles away, "I don't have my flipper in!" Many times I have fallen asleep with it in and gotten up to look at the container I put it in, wondering if the dog ate it, forgetting I had slept in it. My flipper and I have been a good team over the last year. It has enabled me to have a pretty, white, toothy smile. Without it, I look like I lost a big fistfight. Will I miss my flipper? I am sure I will for a minute or two. It seems everything I do reminds me of my mom. My mother had false teeth. She did not have the luxury of seeing a dentist. At an early age she had to get false teeth. It is because of her that I am able to smile today. Her hard work gave me the opportunity to see dentists in my younger years. Each time I smile I will think of her beautiful smile. Thank you, Mom for everything you gave me and have given me. Your gifts still go on and on. xoxoxo

APRIL 9, 2015

I had a dream about my mom this morning. She was lying down and I was standing over her talking to her. We were about five inches apart from one another, her eyes were wide open and she understood everything I was saying to her. I was telling her how much I loved her and did not want her to go. Then the phone rang and woke me up. I was so glad I got to tell her how much I loved her. Was it a dream, or was it real? Who knows? It just was. I also got a letter today from Hospice Plus. They are going to keep in contact with me for the next two years. I found this unbelievably kind. I am continually blessed by the love of so many people. I cannot say enough nice things about Hospice Plus. I met and made so many new friends and they were all placed in mine and mom's life for a reason. Nothing happens by mistake in God's world, nothing. xoxo

APRIL 12, 2015

Since Mom's passing, this is where I sit each morning before I work in her garden. Many of the birdhouses were hers that I brought outside and put in the patio room I decorated. I have integrated her decorations with mine. I sit here and overlook her garden and, of course, she and I have great conversations here. I just get to do all the talking.

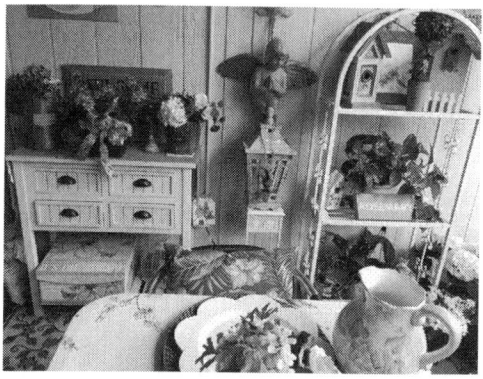

APRIL 13, 2015

For the last three days I have looked like a robot. I have had to move my whole body to look at anyone. It is like my neck stopped working. I could not even drive safely. There was no looking to the left or right. I used my mirrors and prayed. Mindy kept telling me to go get a massage. I finally relented and went tonight. The massage therapist called my neck and upper back a brick. She said they were some of the tightest muscles she had seen. She asked, "Have you had some recent stress?" Since I was naked, under a blanket, and my head was in a hole, I decided to just make a moaning sound, "Mhm." We talked all through the session. She lost her grandfather to Alzheimer's. She was a sweet girl with a sad story. It seems Alzheimer's is affecting more and more people these days. I bet you know someone who has it or someone it is affecting in a negative way. All I can say is this, if you do know a caregiver, please call them and give them a couple of hours to have a break. They sure could use it. Go and visit their loved one. Go visit your loved one. I use to think my mom did not know when I came or left, and maybe she didn't, but even today I wish I had gone more. We do not know the mind of those suffering with this horrible disease, but we do know the mind of a caregiver and they are hurting. Give them some love, and that means some time away from those they are caring for. By the way, my neck feels so much better. I knew you were wondering. xoxoxoo

APRIL 14, 2015

Today has been one of those tough days. No rhyme or reason. I just realized it had been a month and three days since Mom passed. My mother had Doves and Purple Martins in her yard. I could not even go into her house for about six months after we put her in a facility, it was too sad. The following Spring I finally went in, and the birds she loved had taken over. I began the tedious job of cleaning everything up and trying not to disturb her babies. They came back the following year. The day she passed; I came to her garden and a Dove was on the fence. I thought it was early in the year to see it there. Unfortunately, the pair has never returned and none of the Purple Martins have returned either since her passing. This truly saddens me. I was sitting in her garden today looking at the empty Purple Martin house, and then looking at the empty Dove nest I had carefully taken care of for the past two years. They are gone, she is gone. Maybe they went to Heaven to be with her, *yes that must be it* I told myself. When I focus on where she is and not on my sadness, I am able to let go of my pain. She and her Doves, and her Purple Martins are up in Heaven. What a beautiful thought. If I focus on Heaven and her happiness then I can be happy and not so sad.

The Dove came to me to say "Goodbye"

The same Dove who nested outside

He no longer comes to this nest

He only came to tell me Goodbye

On the same day Rosie died.

He flew to Heaven to build his nest there

He wanted to be with her just like before

The Doves she so much adored.

Rosemary's Garden has a plan

All the birds and flowers understand

We are only here for a short stay

Heaven will set us all free

We will all be Redeemed...heart emoticon heart emoticon heart emoticon

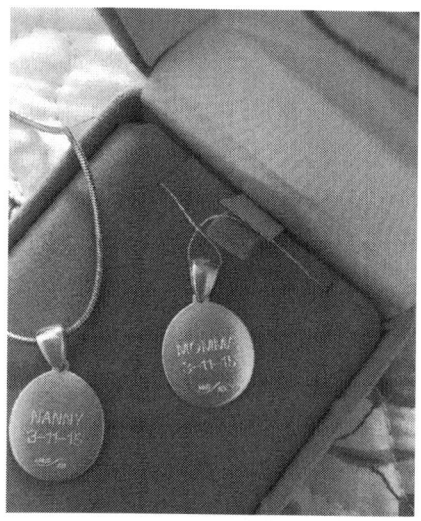

APRIL 15, 2015

Wow, I feel like such a dweeb. I took Mindy her charm today. She looked at me and said, "This one is Jane's, and mine is supposed to say Nanny." "HUH?" was my answer. Then it clicked in my brain; we had ordered three different names to be engraved on each thumbnail, Nanny for Mindy, Momma for me and Rosie for Jane. We each called her by those names. I thought they all said "Rosie" because that is what everyone else called my mom. When I came home I looked at the other ones still in the box and sure enough I found mine, with Momma on it, and Mindy's with Nanny.

I don't know how a name can make such a difference but it does. I will cherish it much more, now that it says, Momma. xoxo

APRIL 16, 2015

I spoke with my publisher today. I am going to add a whole new chapter to my book, "*Fading Image*." It will be about the beginning of mine and Mom's journey together, my reason for getting involved so heavily in her life, her disease and ultimately getting Legal Guardianship. I am so excited about getting so close to the end. My publisher told me not to rush it. No problem with that these days. I have so much information in my head and so much I want to share. I surely do not want others to make any of the mistakes I made. I also want all available resources out there for other to access. Not only will it be our story, but also I want it to be a book of constant resource for others. A book full of laughter, answers and especially one of hope. When you finish reading "Fading Image," you will have hope and see that my mom and I, although we had our struggles, came out victorious in every area of our journey. Please know too, that family, friends AND Facebook friends, have always helped me and mom along our journey and given me some of the best ideas for my book. xoox

APRIL 20, 2015
A day with Kenady, Mom and me.

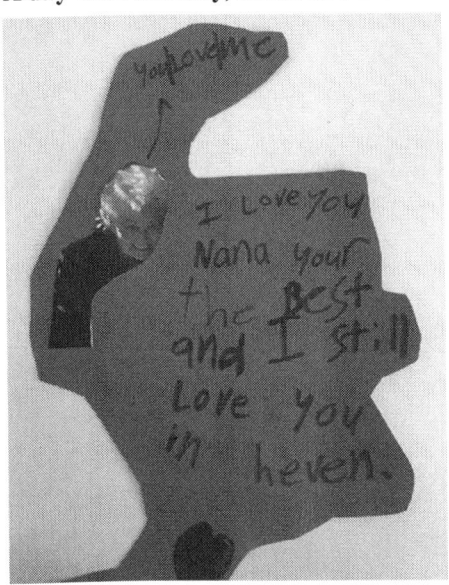

APRIL 22, 2015

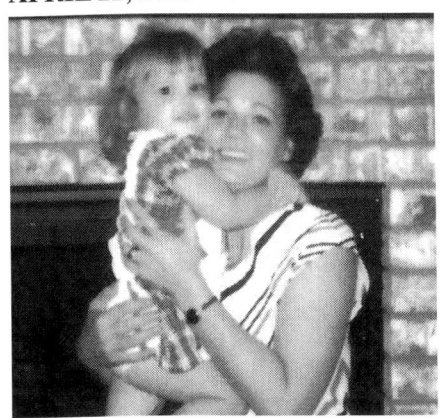

It was one of those tough days today. As I was getting ready for bed tonight, I went outside and saw a bag on the garage floor. I looked in it and there were more pictures. As I flipped through them I found this picture. It's as though Mom always sends me a picture when I am really missing her. Here is one of my two greatest loves, Mom and my Mindy

APRIL 23, 2015

Yesterday, when I went by Moms after being with Dawnie, my hairdresser whom I love and adore, I was going through her mail. There was a sympathy card inside. It contained the most thoughtful memories of my mom. Karen, the mail carrier, had motioned to me to come back outside years before, and shared with me that she felt something strange was going on with Mom. Mom was not engaging with her like she used to. So, I made sure I kept Karen up to date on Mom's condition. The only reason Karen was not at the funeral was because she was out of town. In her card she wrote of times she and Mom laughed, and the gifts Mom left her every holiday. Mom and Murray were the kind of people who became friends with the trash collectors, every neighbor and especially Karen. In the rush of our everyday lives I think we forget those who do a service for us. It is their job some would say, but it is still doing a service for us. I remember when I was doing my nursing and a patient brought me a handmade gift, a book, candy, card or anything, I always felt so loved and special. How hard is it to tell someone they are doing a "good job?" My mom and Murray had the right idea. Treat everyone with love and respect, and they will never forget you for your kindness. Karen did not forget Mom, and her card clearly stated as such. When I write her back today, I will make sure she knows, Mom adored her too. xoxo

APRIL 25, 2015

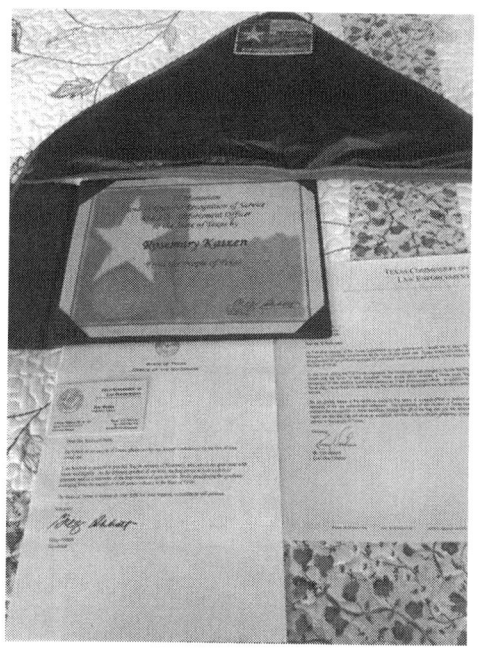

Yesterday I received a huge box in the mail. It contained a Texas state flag. A letter from Greg Abbot, the Governor of Texas, and two certificates. I read the letter from the Texas Commissioner of Law Enforcement, sending condolences for my loss and for my loved one's sacrifice and service to the citizens of the State of Texas. She went on to say they are greatly aware of the sacrifices made by the family of a peace officer in dealing with the demands of the law enforcement profession. In the last sentence the Executive Director said her hopes were that the flag would be a positive reminder of the profound greatness of Rosemary's service to the people of Texas. The letter from Gregg Abbott stated the same and even more. He thanked me for my support, commitment and patience. As a child, a teenager and an adult child of a police officer, I always considered it a privilege to be even remotely associated with the DPD, and I always will. I can't ever remember a time when I did not think of a police officer as someone who put his or her life on the line every day. My mother carried a gun to work. I knew it was not a play gun. I knew it had real bullets and was for protection for her and for others. She carried it in a purse, but she still had it on her to be used if needed. I see the recent stories and problems going on all around me with peace officers and I am biased to say the least. Most of my life I was associated with "police officers" and I can honestly say they were, and are, all heroes to me. It is not a job I would want, but I am definitely grateful there are those who do want the job. Thank God for them, past and present.

APRIL 25, 2015

I only wish she had known just how awesome she was and still is. Now, maybe she does. My mother was as respectful as she was beautiful. Thank you to Governor Greg Abbott, Texas Commissioner Kim Vickers, and the 77th Texas Legislature House Bill 815. I will treasure every piece of certification sent to me and also the Texas state flag.

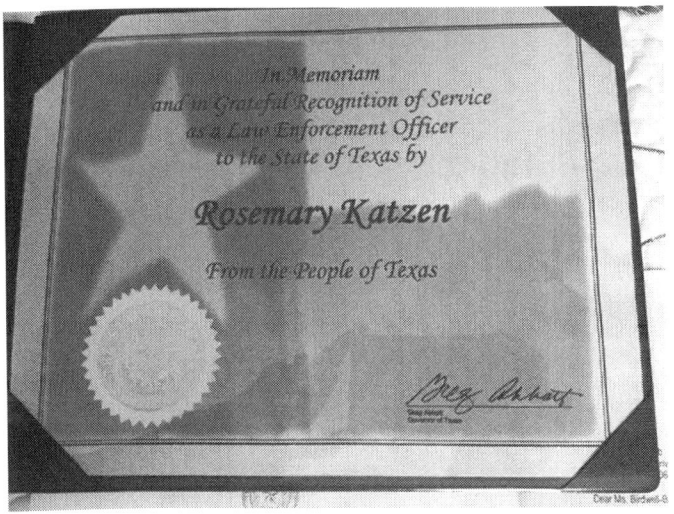

MAY 1, 2015

My beautiful friends...guys included
Friends are like the perfect shade of lipstick
It makes your face glow when it is applied
Friends are like the most delicious dessert
You have ever tasted or tried
Friends are like that perfect pillow you lay your head upon
It cradles the head and you're fast asleep before your first yawn
Friends are like a mother when you were a small child
She held you, told you how wonderful you were
Answered all calls, and turned those tears into smiles.

Friends are the promises that life goes on and on
The grace of God places them there
So you don't ever have to be alone.

With Mother's Day only being a little over a week away, I started thinking how all of my friends have helped me so much in the last few months. Dealing with the loss of Mom. Although I no longer have my mother, I have been loved and mothered by many friends. What would I have done without you guys? I would hate to have to imagine that. The kindness and gentleness have been overwhelming. It is like I have many mothers, sisters and friends all rolled into one. What can you say about friends? Everything and more. Thank you for loving me during this tough time. You are all unbelievable in your own way. xoxox

MAY 2, 2015

The last few weeks have been a turning point for me. I see how God has had a plan in my life, my daughter's life, even my mom's life. Everything happened exactly when it was supposed to. It is like my mom knew when it was time to leave us and that is when she left. When I think back on all those days I was so fearful of her disease, the trials and tribulations we all went through, it seemed so insurmountable and yet we made it through. I see how God was with me the whole time, even though sometimes I felt all alone. I was never alone. If I can share one thing it is this, God is there, especially in those moments you feel most alone. You will look back and see that you were not alone. You were loved by him every step of the way!
God's undeniable love
It's not until the thunderstorm eases
The lightning lessens and the storm ceases
I could clearly see your plan
Though I trudged thru a mire of frightening steps
You were always there to hold my hand
I ran and hid, denying at times
Any love for me at all
So you held me even tighter
So I could not further fall
As I look behind me...
I clearly see your beautifully laid out plan.
And because of all of it ...
I will never have to question

Your love for me, ever again.

MAY 7, 2015

As Mother's Day approaches I am inundated with how women have changed the world in so many ways. I spoke with a Verizon representative yesterday, he was a male and the subject turned to Mom's. He had just recently lost his mom too. His voice immediately changed and became quieter and gentler as he spoke of her. He said, "You never get over losing a mother." I truly felt his pain. Whenever I speak to anyone who has lost a mom, no matter how long it has been, they are still experiencing great loss. Later in the conversation I spoke to a female representative and she helped me through the steps with my router. She was quick-witted, carefully explanatory and honestly, I did not feel stupid as she went over the steps with me. I was able to get my problem solved. This was after I had worked with two other guys and could not get this done. The other night when I went for my sleep study, a gentleman came into the room to explain the steps to me. I felt uncomfortable and was hoping it would be a female instead. I did not feel that calm, easy feeling I do with another female. In 2012 when I had to call a Rowlett police officer to assist in some abuse my mother was going through, I actually prayed for a female officer to arrive. Lo and behold, one did. We have been friends from that day forward and I still think of her as part of the overall plan that God had, to get my mom to safety. I have a female physician I trust with all my medical needs. I believe she and I are personal friends today, too. Don't get me wrong, I love and adore men, I just think there is something innately placed in a woman that makes her more in tune to the needs of one's heart, mind and spirit. Why do we love our mother's so much? I believe it is because they are so full of love, understanding, warmth, and a peace that passes all understanding. God did not make men and women the same. Women are not only strong when we need to be, but we are also intuitive to others pain and we want to make it better. We are Mommies to not only our children, but to the neighbor's kids, our fur babies and even our plants. We just have that need to nurture. It is no wonder we love our mothers so much. I don't just like my female friends, I love them. My mother taught me love by loving me. She was a great role model. My mother lost her own mother at a very young age and her mother was sick for many years before she died. My mother did not have the best role model due to her own mother's disease. She must have done something right when it came to loving me because I sure do love her. You can't learn love from any schoolbook. Thank you God for mothers and for making me a woman who can love so easily. xoxo

MAY 10, 2015

I received a gift from Heaven, my mom's purple martin house had one door that had come loose over the years. I kept thinking I was seeing something in the empty hole. I looked closer and, of all things, she has a pair of Doves in one slot of the Purple Martin house. That is going to be some tight space when baby doves are born; they have four at a time. I felt this was a gift from my mom to me. It is just like my mom to find the smallest space but make the out of it.

I love you Mom, Happy Mother's Day. Thanks for your gift. xoxoo

MAY 12, 2015

I am not a movie critic but I do know more than I want to know about Alzheimer's. Here is my take on the movie, "Still Alice." The movie was very good. Although, I think I saw it too soon after losing my mom. It was very depressing for me. The reason being is that it showed me just how scared Mom probably was when she had the first signs of her disease. If, or when, you watch the movie, don't feel as though they dramatized the acting when it came to the disease. They did not. They sugar coated it in my opinion. My meaning is, they did not show just how devastating it could be to the sufferer or the caregivers. But, I can understand why. You don't want to leave a movie wanting to vomit. If you get a chance, see the movie. You will get an understanding of what an Alzheimer's sufferer goes through. My mom and I had problems when she first got the disease. I thought she was mad at me and I could not understand why. Unfortunately, I pulled back. I wish I had it to do all over again. In those days, little was said about the disease and even less was known. I hope in some small way I made that time up to her. Hopefully, we will find a cure to this horrific disease. Be open to watching for signs from your parents and loved ones. Don't assume they are mad when it could just be fear, or their brain is out of kilter. We are all in this together, all of us.

MAY 13, 2015

Just had a wonderful visit with a friend I made while she and her other "earthly angels" took care of Mom. Hospice was so good to mom, my family and me those last few months. Katrina DeAnn Montenegro, you, Amanda and the others will always have a special place in my heart. I am so glad we were able to continue our friendship long past the passing of my mom. Thank you for the beautiful cross and other little gifts today. You forgot your mint! That's a good excuse to come back and see me, and visit Rosemary's Garden again. xoxoox

MAY 16, 2015

I just finished cleaning out the closet at Mom's house. It had to be done for the ADT guys to install the new security system. I found a book we thought was lost. It is called "Reflections from a Mother's Heart." It is actually a journal a mother writes in and answers questions about her own life. One of the questions in the book ask,

"What is your most vivid memory of being pregnant?"

My mother's answer, "I threw up all the time. I was so sick. If I went anywhere I had to carry a bucket, it lasted nine months. I like to feel you kick. I was just a baby myself. I was the last kid to be born so I had never been around a younger brother or sister. I knew nothing about what to do. You were so beautiful and a very good baby."

Mindy has told me of two dreams she has had about Mom and Dad has told me of one. I kept wondering why Mom does not come to me in dreams, but she does come to me. She comes to me in pictures I find. She comes to me in journals I find that we were sure were lost; she comes to me by way of the doves in backyard. She has never left me.

Writing is so essential; it goes on and on even when we are gone. My mother speaks to me even now. Please take time to write in a journal for your loved ones. One day they may need to hear from you the same way I needed to hear from her.

I love you Momma. xoxoox

JUNE 2, 2015

My mother and her deceased husband, Murray Katzen, are still blessing me on a daily basis. At least once a week I will hear from someone who has heard about Mom's passing. They will reflect on something about her, and then also something about Murray. Just yesterday an old friend of Murray's, who was an attorney, spoke to Mindy about how Mom had shown him her pistol, as she called it, and told him she never left home without it. He went on to tell Mindy how he adored Mom and Murray. I saw my grief counselor yesterday; he had the pleasure of meeting my mom in her latter days of Alzheimer's. He, through me, had gotten to know her history. We both gave thought yesterday on what an awesome woman she was. I often felt such sadness thinking once she passed I would never get to talk about how great I thought my mom was. I wouldn't get to brag on her again. I realized yesterday, that memories live on forever, and when you are someone like my mom was, people just do not forget you. I think in the world today we focus way too much on negativity, how others have wronged us, our terrible plight in life and so on. I want to spend my days looking toward the things I have to be grateful. I am so grateful I still have my memory so that I can reflect on my mom and also all those who still hold me up when I feel so sad at times. Life is so good, it truly is. Thank you God for the gift of family and friends. They lift me out of the shadows of sadness into the light of happiness and love. xoxoxo

JUNE 9, 2015

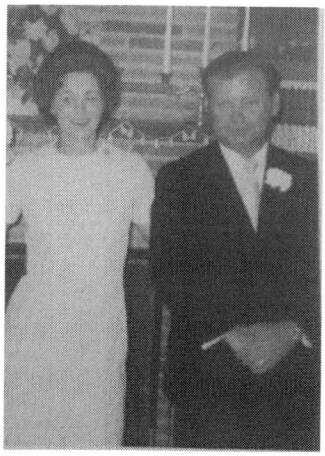

My daughter went to visit the family of her deceased father yesterday. Her dad's stepsister was there and had pictures of mine and James' wedding. She was able to take this picture with her cell phone camera. This is my mom and dad when they were still together. I think they were in their thirties. My parents were always such a beautiful couple. This picture makes me miss my mom even more. She was a great woman and an even better policewoman. I am so proud of her and her 33 years of service with the DPD. xoxo

JUNE 15, 2015

Here it is, so close to Father's Day and I am missing my mom more than ever. I have done really well the last few weeks. Then someone will call and ask how I am doing and the water works come. Maybe I allow myself, at that time, to actually think of her. Today I thought of the times I probably hurt her in some of the stupid things I did or said. When you are young you think you know everything. I moved away once and although it was best for me, I think it just about killed her. I know it must have hurt her deeply and to this day I regret it. I hope in some small way I made it up to her when I moved back to Dallas. I think sometimes if there are 100 people who love us and one who does not, we chase after that one who does not. We do everything we can to get that one person to love us and we ignore the other 99 who already adore us. We just cannot understand why one person would not love us, too. Sometimes we need to focus on what is right in front of us. My mom use to always tell me this, but did I listen? Probably not. My mom was a great woman, a great mom, and a great friend. I hope she can see just how much I miss her. I hope I live up to all of her expectations of me. I love you and miss you so much Momma. xoxo

JUNE 19, 2015

In the last week I have had three people contact me with inquiries about a loved one that has similar symptoms of Alzheimer's. Some have a loved one who is experiencing the last chapter of their lives. Sometimes I am on my way out the door and once I was in the tub when I got a text. Other times I am down and in my own thoughts. To me, it does not matter if I am knee deep in everything, I will take that text, that call, that inquiry. Whenever I was in need, during those caregiving days with my mom, I was thankful for every call, every touch, and every text answered for me. Some of the most loving and kind people I have met, I met in the nursing field and through Hospice. People like this go through school and college to learn the medical part of helping others, but that genuine "love and caring" is just part of who they are. If I can help one person suffer less anxiety, less fear, and less loss in their own journey with their loved one, then my suffering becomes less. I can't explain it. It is like the sad memories of those days with my mother become happier memories if I use them to help another. We are all in this together, us silly humans.

JULY 11, 2015

I am going on a trip in a few days. I have not been anywhere in over seven years, where I was not worried about my mom, and constantly monitoring my phone. Last year we all went to Port Aransas and took fur babies. This year we will have to leave them since we are going by plane. I travel very little. I visited the awesome place where I take my dogs to see the vet. I was going to board them there. When I saw where they would be for eight days I started crying like a big, baby. I am sure they thought I was crazy. They were all super kind. I called my daughter and said, "I am not going, go without me on the trip." I was serious. I have so much going on at Mom's house anyway, so much contracting work. There were so many "maybes" and "ifs," and this and that's. It was just not going to work. My daughter texted me, the contractor called me, another contractor emailed me, and it all fell into place. I am going and my fur babies will be able to be home and taken care of by a family friend who lives a few miles away. Someone I did not even think would be available. Some way or another I felt my mom was involved in all this. I think she would want me to go. She loved to travel, loved it. Thank you to my beautiful daughter who was there for me at this time and has been there for most of my grief process that I am continuing to work through.

JULY 14, 2015

As they did work around my mom's house today, and I was speaking with the contractor, I just started crying. I could feel my mom standing right next to me. She was smiling as she watched the work being done. I asked the contractor if I could put some of her things in a box under the concrete they would be pouring. He put his arm around me and said, "Do whatever you need to do and I will take care of it and we will put it in a special place." I felt a little silly but he seemed to totally understand. I was so proud of my mom when she was alive and I always got great pleasure in telling everyone about all her attributes. I was going to miss doing that. I realize I still can share about her. The awesome thing is, everyone has a mom, and everyone seems to understand my love, admiration and feelings of loss. I will never forget you Momma! <3

A small sample of sweet fruits

A peek of breathless views

A wisp of flowered bouquets

A whisper of the cool breeze

All the Serenity....

I just wished to see you in my dreams.

You, on the other hand, wanted me to see Heaven-

Through the peephole of Hawaii.

I see you and God EVERYWHERE Mom. xoxo

JULY 29, 2015

When we got in yesterday the house was still intact, the babies were well and work was still being done around the house. I lost a few plants but those can be replaced. Boomer, our family friend Tristen, stayed at the house while we were on vacation. All in all, things could not have been better thanks to him. I noticed a box on the counter. I remembered one of my cousins said I might be getting something from her. My mom had seven older brother and sisters. I opened the box and inside was a beautiful afghan in pink and white. I love pink. The card stated, "The afghan is for you, I made it in memory of your mom, my aunt." She also included a cookbook she and her husband personally had a hand in making for the church they attend in Nevada. I received so many cards from cousins when Mom passed, most stating she was their favorite aunt. In Hawaii, I was able to leave so much of my heartache there and come home to so much love. I know God has more in store for me. I see and feel my mother's handi-work in all these things that are happening in my life these days. A Mom just never stops taking care of those she loves, love has the longest extension cord. Reaching and loving you from Heaven is a piece of cake when it comes to a mom, take it from me, I know. xooxo

JULY 31, 2015

I just had my mom and Murray's peach tree cut down. I remember all the years we ate peaches from that tree. I remember all the peaches she gave away to the neighbors. This spring it was covered in baby peaches. More proliferate than ever before. Then all the torrential rains came and it died within a couple of weeks. I have to say she went out with a bang. I feel such a loss. I know it has more to do with so many losses in my life this year, not only my mom but so many of my friends have had losses, too. It is just a tree, but it is a tree that held so many memories. When we lose those we love, we often think, what could I have done differently? God gives us such a heart for all living things. Although it hurts to feel such love and loss, I still think it is a good thing to simply feel. xoxo Thank you God for giving me the heart to feel sad when a tree dies, another one of your creations. <3<3

I Love You A Bushel And A Peck And A Folder That Weighs Five Pounds And Three Ounces

When I first started keeping records for Mom, I kept a couple of sheets of paper in a thin, green folder. I think I found it somewhere around the house. It had been in one of the drawers and probably had belonged to one of the grandkids at one time. Harry, my counselor, suggested I start keeping records of everything. He would always say, all the records might come in handy one day, what sage advice. The first court visit we had was an emergency try for guardianship. It is virtually impossible to get this type of guardianship. If a person is fed, has a roof over their head, clothes on their back and a court appointed attorney ad litem, then you have a 90% chance of not gaining guardianship, even if they want it. Guardianship takes away every right an adult has. You can no longer vote, drive, or make any independent decisions. You give your rights over to another person. You cease to exist as yourself, quite frankly. My mom was deemed mentally incompetent from tests, but with what little bit of knowledge she had left, she did not want to admit she could not be an independent person. Also, if you are being told by someone that the person trying to gain guardianship of you is the enemy, you can bet you do not trust that person to be in control of you and all your decisions. Mindy and I were in for the fight of our lives. So, the little green folder grew and grew.

After losing the Emergency Guardianship we were devastated, but told we could go after Permanent Guardianship and not to lose hope. We would just have more time to get all of our ducks in a row. Of course I was devastated thinking I was leaving her to her own devices in the meantime. I had no control over her medications, her doctor visits or even if she saw a doctor. I had no control over my mom at all. I knew she was not being properly cared for. She needed constant care and I knew she needed Mindy and me, two people who adored her. That weekend my daughter and grandkids decided to go out of town. I got a call from the court investigator. I returned her call, and she explained to me she would investigate me, and Mom's current living conditions. She would then turn in her report, and the report of a court appointed doctor who also specialized in mental illness testing. After this investigation it would be her determination who should have guardianship of my mom. I was ecstatic. Here was my chance to rescue my mom. There was no doubt in my mind who would be awarded guardianship. The facts were there for anyone to see. I knew the truth would shine through. I just never knew how slow the court process was, or how hard a court appointed attorney ad litem fights for the person who is impaired. Even when it is clearly a better choice for them to give up their rights. I guess we all have a right to be independent. I just think this defies logic to some degree. But, the law is the law. Mindy and I **abided by every law**; this is what Mom taught us both.

The flat green folder began to grow bigger and bigger, fatter and fatter. After the phone call with the court investigator, the writer in me decided the best way for her to understand what was going on was to *write* about Mom. I had to tell her a little about Mom, her past, our past. I took pictures of the railroad tracks where she had been stuck for many hours. I made a copy of the email I had sent to the Argyle police officer and his return email to me, which detailed how he found Mom in her car on the tracks at 3:00 AM that morning, with the train whistle blowing. He had saved her. She had been missing for 15 hours. Yes, these are things that needed to be told. Pictures are worth a thousand words. I had the pictures and I would include the words. The folder contained medical doctor's reports, hundreds of them. I had gone and asked all of the doctors for their reports. Since I had been taking her to her visits, I was able to get the records. I put attorney receipts in the folder, and any and every thing that had to do with Mom. I was determined to win guardianship of her. I would save her. During this time she professed to hate me when we were in court, or she was served intermittently. Other times she was fine around me. I was no longer afraid of making people angry. I was on a mission to save her and no matter what toll it took on me mentally, physically or spiritually, I would save her. There were so many doctor visits, so much time in between. I would grow weary of what was taking place with her. But the folder grew and grew. I was being *empowered* by *empowering her*. The court date was coming up for guardianship and I was getting very worried. What would I do if I lost? How could I reconcile myself to the fact that I had not done enough to save her? How would I live with myself? My daughter was out of town and I was swimming in her pool a few nights before the court date. I was on one of her floats, and to the right of me I saw a shooting star. Immediately after seeing the star I felt as though God's arms totally enveloped me. I could hear Him say that everything would be ok. He would take care of me and of Mom. This was the first time I felt true peace for mom. I knew, at that moment, I would get guardianship of my mom. On the next court date, mom, at this time, did not even understand what was going on. She just smiled at me from the other side of the room. Maybe down, deep inside, she was glad but afraid to show it. She did still have to live with *him*. I would work on taking care of that next.

After I was awarded guardianship of Mom, I would like to say things were perfect, but they were not. I kept records of everything that took place. Adult Protective Services would come in handy during those next few months as did caregivers. God never places anyone in your life by mistake, never.

In August of 2012, my mom was totally free of all dangers surrounding her, albeit the Alzheimer's. We no longer had to fear any outside forces. A few months later she was free to become as close to "normal" as she could be. She began a road back to a healthier Rosemary. Her skin began to look better. She gained some weight, she got her color back, and her thinned hair began to thicken up over time. She laughed again. The right kind of medication, love and care can help an Alzheimer's sufferer do better. We had her almost two and a half more years.

During this time, and for almost a year, my mom and I made up for lost time. We found one another again, and our love and admiration grew stronger than ever. I found things in her home I had never seen before. I found my mom for who she really was. She was a hero. She was a pioneer for women all over America during the 1950's and beyond. She fulfilled her dream. She made something of herself. Boy, did she! I still have that green folder. I still use it even today. I use it to look things up when I need information about her. I will most likely pass it down from one generation to the next. I have her newspaper clippings from the Dallas Morning News, even some of her old pay stubs from the DPD. I am so glad I made the folder. These are things I wrote about her and kept, starting in 2010. Things others wrote about her too.

I weighed the folder before I wrote this chapter. The weight was five pounds and three ounces. My mom use to always say, she loved me a bushel, and a peck and a hug around the neck. Well, I can say I love her the same, plus a five pound, three ounce green folder.

I did it all for my mom. I would do it all again, every single solitary page.

There Is A Pink Elephant In The room? Wow, There Sure Is!

There were days my mom would call me and ask me why I had taken her panties out of her room. Why did I steal her lipstick? I had not been in her house in over six months. She had been isolated from everyone. I got calls from her accusing me of using her charge cards. It was not me using them; I had no access to her credit cards. In her mind, this was her truth. Some of this I am sure was due to her lack of medications, or the meds being given incorrectly. Some of this was malnutrition and some was the first stages of Alzheimer's. In those days, when she called I tried my best to reason with her. I tried to explain that I could not get into her house; I did not have a key. I could not use her credit cards, and did not have access to them. Then she would call me names, names I had never been called by her, before. I would spend the rest of the day confused, sad and wondering what was going on with my mom. I felt totally helpless. I can't tell you how many times I cried after our phone calls. I took it all personally.

After I got Adult Protective Services involved, the abusive behavior from her got worse. There were more phone calls and more accusations. The mother I adored, revered and loved all my life had turned into someone I felt had abandoned me and turned into a creature from the deep Lagoon of Hell. So many times I felt like just giving up, but this little voice inside my head kept saying, *this is not your mother speaking, help her!* It would have been far easier to walk away. I only suspected the fight I had before me.

When you feel a loved one is in need of saving, you don't have to hear that voice twice to take action. I am her daughter; I could not ever forget that.

I soon learned years later, once she was in a memory care unit, that she would tell me many strange and wonderful things. One day she shared that a rattlesnake had bitten her. I looked at the wound. I kissed it and told her to stay away from the woods. She kissed me back. Another time she spoke of her deceased father coming and visiting her. Someone in the room was aghast and I said, "Oh, how sweet Mom, he must really love you." She often asked me why he did not come more often or where was he. These are the times I told her a "love lie." I used to get so upset when she would talk about seeing her dead parents in the facility until my counselor shared with me that it was a good thing. This meant she felt safe where she was if they were in the same facility.

There was no sense in arguing with her, it made no difference. It was her truth. That Alzheimer's brain was working its mojo on her. Was I going to make it worse and argue with her? No, not for a minute.

Don't argue with an Alzheimer's sufferer. If they tell you there is a pink elephant in the room, then go along with it. If they say someone came through the window, believe them. Of course, you can check it out and when, or if, you find it is not true, remember it is true to them. Change the subject if they accuse you of things. You cannot change their mind. My mom thought I took her panties, no matter how many times I told her I was not in her house. It is so hard to hear some of the hurtful things a loved one may say to you. Just keep telling yourself, it is not them talking, it is Alzheimer's. This disease is rude, cunning, baffling and takes no prisoners.

Love Lies

I hated lying to my mom. I was raised to tell her the truth.

There comes a time when you have to lie to the Alzheimer sufferer. It feels awful and you feel like you are doing them a real disservice. How can I lie to my parent like this? I am blatantly being deceiving. This was one of those things that bothered me the most. Even writing about it now makes me sad.

There are times you will have to lie. The times you take your loved one to a memory care unit and them to their room. This is the hardest trip you will make. Before leaving, your loved one will most likely ask, are you leaving me here? That look on their face, the sadness in their eyes is devastating, and heartbreaking.

Love lie number one: "I am leaving you here so they can check you out. It is a new type of hospital. Don't you love your room? You have your own special care. I will see you tomorrow." Your loved one is scared to death. The sheer fact of having Alzheimer's is scary enough. Do you really want to explain the "truth" to them? Do you want to say I have placed you in memory care unit and you won't be living at home anymore? No, of course not. Tell them what will make them happy. Tell them what will make them feel safe. Lie, lie, and lie! Make it the best LOVE LIE you can come up with. They will not remember or know that you did not tell them the truth. I promise.

What the Alzheimer sufferer wants is to feel loved and safe. They are petrified. Hold them when they are afraid. Don't rationalize with them, they do not understand. Don't argue with them, they do not understand. Tell them you will protect them. You will always be there for them, always.

This is not a lie, this is love.

Predators in the Alzheimer's World

I have always been one of those people who tell it like it is. In other words, I am going to be very honest with you. Check out everyone who will be around your Alzheimer sufferer.

Mom had been diligent about certain things, her Prenuptial Agreement, her Will, her Power of Attorney and so on. When you have parties that ignore all these court documents you must play "catch up," "reset," "replay," and so on. You hire an attorney to enforce laws that should have been followed to begin with. First, you have to prove inappropriate behavior and then after months you can begin the beginning. I think what I am trying to express here to everyone reading this about your loved one is this, you must watch those *closest to your loved one*.

Have you ever watched a crime show about someone missing, or a crime-taking place? Most crimes are committed by a family member or someone we know closely. It is a sad fact.

Watch your loved one, watch for signs of abuse from any and from everyone. Get all the appropriate forms filled out. Don't be afraid to ask your parent if they have a Will. If so, who has the Power of Attorney; whom have they designated as their Medical Power of Attorney? Of course, these are hard questions but if these things are not taken care of – you will spend thousands of dollars and years as I did taking care of this after the fact.

Watch banks, they are notorious for abusing the elderly. The elderly believe banks can be thoroughly trusted. They are told by someone they have been banking with for years that their money would be much better off in this annuity or this money market. When the mind starts going they will trust others before they trust you. Remember, the mind is no longer their own. It belongs to Alzheimer's now.

Be wary of new love relationships. Men and women prey on the elderly when they know they have limited abilities. Many relationships have been made in church

Heaven and ended in court Hell. There are predators everywhere

When picking a memory care unit ask for references from doctors and from other caregivers. Get many and then some. Go at nighttime, because this is the best time to check. I will write more on this in another chapter.

Am I saying be wary of everyone? You better believe it. Your parent is not the same parent or loved one you once knew. Would you expect a five-year-old to make a rational, informative decision? Of course not. They trust everyone and most likely believe what everyone tells them.

Your loved one is just like a child at times. Protect them. Remember you are leaving a five-year-old in the care of all these people. You don't let a five-year-old drive, make changes on accounts at banks, or dispense themselves their own medications. This is Alzheimer's, beware!

I did Not Recognize Her Anymore

The last few months when I would go and see Mom I could barely recognize her. Where was my mom? Not only was she no longer the woman I knew, she did not even look the same. Her hair was not brushed, her clothes had food on them, her fingernails were all different lengths, the polish was chipped, and sometimes she was barefooted.

I would think to myself, I had just polished her nails a few days ago, what had happened. I had sent her to the beauty parlor at the center, what was going on with her hair? She smelled like she had soiled her pants and sometimes she had.

One day I watched her walk to her recliner, pull down her pants and her underwear and start to relieve herself in her chair. I yelled, "NO, Mom, not there!" She quickly stopped. I ran to where she was and directed her to the restroom. She did not even shut the bathroom door. She had no modesty left; she did not even care who saw her use the restroom. Many times she would see me cry for her. She would get a sad, concerned look on her face and then her attention would be focused somewhere else. I was dying inside for her.

There were times I would rush to brush her hair, even try and curl it for her. I would put lipstick on her, a little cologne and change her clothes. The first year or so she would let me, towards the end, she just wanted to sleep and be left alone. One time in the last year I saw her look in the mirror, I could tell she did not even recognize herself. She mussed her hair a little and then looked away. It was like the image was too hard for her to accept. It was that day that I decided I would no longer post pictures of her on Facebook. I would not do that to her. I knew she would want it that way.

My mom was the most beautiful woman. She had dark hair and hazel eyes. As she grew older her eyes lightened. She had skin like Snow White. I remember my mom never having one blemish. She was always smiling. My mom was always so slim. She was modeling on the side while she was doing her police work. My mother was all that and a bag of chips. To see the way she was now was devastating to me. I did not even know this woman. This was not my mom on the outside, but inside she was still there. I could feel her I just could not see her.

My mom and I got closer those last two years. Closer than we had ever been in our whole adult lives. She worked so much of the time while I was growing up, but I always knew Mom loved me. As a child I would sit between her legs on the floor, while she pin curled my hair every night, whether I liked it or not. We were a team, Mom and I. I put her on the highest pedestal and there she stayed the majority of my life. I visited her at the police department, invited her to my school, showed her off to my friends and somewhere along the line we lost one another over the years, until she became very sick and needed me again. Never did I know how much I would need her needing me.

Here she was depending on me for EVERYTHING. I was her decision maker, her memory, her bodyguard and her defender. So, how could I let any more pictures be taken of her? This was not my mom. This was a picture of the disease of Alzheimer's. Why would I want to show off the "monster?" I hated what it had done to her. I would ask Mindy and others to not post any more pictures of mom, the reason being, it was not her anymore.

The essence of Mom was gone and could not be photographed. You could ask me about Mom and I could tell you, because I knew her better than anyone. Yes, me, her daughter. I knew who she was, what she was really like. This person you saw now, this was not my mom. I grieved every day for the mom who was already gone. I had to lose her all over again. Every single, solitary day.

Sometimes I wished God would take her. I knew it had always been her biggest fear to have a mental illness. Was this what she feared? Of course it was. It was being incapacitated. It was not knowing what you were capable of, it was depending on others. It was being mentally incompetent. It was a way of allowing others to take advantage of you. This had always been her biggest fear. How had she known? She had asked Mindy and I for years to promise her we would not allow her to live in some vegetative state, she had filled out a directive specifically stating as such. She had filled out so many forms, she knew in some way something like this was going to happen. Her fears had become a reality. Her own mother had suffered from schizophrenia. Mom did not have that disease, but something more debilitating maybe. One never knows how any mental illness will affect someone or other members of a family. However, I do know this, secrets keep us sick. My mom kept her fear a secret from her family for years. This fear probably plagued her most of her life. God only knows how these fears affected her in the long run. All I can hope and pray for is that she never knew how sick she became, that is the one saving grace of Alzheimer's. You don't know how sick you become or what you do. Thank you God for that.

Alzheimer's Is Not
A Disease For Sissies

My mom was definitely a survivor. My cousin and I often joke with one another about being Dedman girls. We say we can be tough, because we have the Dedman blood in our body. My mom was one of those tough Dedman girls. She was born to Rosa and Arch P. Dedman; an Arkansas farming family, barely making ends meet. My mom survived being born as the baby of eight other children. She survived having a mother with Schizophrenia, she survived the loss of a sibling, and she survived the great depression, although it would shape the rest of her life. She survived having a baby when she herself was a baby. She survived one of the first police academy training's. She survived a divorce, the death of a spouse, and she also survived abuse from someone she thought loved and cared for her. The one thing she could never overcome was her Alzheimer's Disease.

In the beginning of her disease there were few of us who really knew something was wrong. I was one of them. My mom was a survivor, so much so that she even fought Alzheimer's with a knee jerk reaction. It was just in her makeup. There were people that would go visit her at the Memory Care Unit and call me after and tell me how in the beginning of the conversation she acted so normal, so herself. Some of us have a tendency to ask an Alzheimer sufferer, "Do you remember this or so and so?" Most will say, yes. They may even think they do. They can carry on a full fledge conversation and appear to be as normal as you or I. Just don't ask them to give you change for a dollar or remember what your telephone number was, or even who the president is. It depends on what part of the brain is impaired. Our brains have different structures that control different emotions, feelings and motor skills. It all depends on where the damage is. I am trying to make this as easily explainable as one can.

My mother had social skills she had acquired through life. She was on automatic pilot. You don't have the experiences someone like Mom had, and not learn how to cope. She had learned most of her life to make excuses for her own mother's disease. It was ingrained in her.

During my years with her at the Memory Care Unit, I grew closer and closer to her. I was her memory, and her voice when she had none. I was her bodyguard and defender. All of us who have loved ones with this disease can relate. You not only want to take up for your loved one, but you want to fight the disease at the same time. You want a cure, a pill, compassion, but you mainly want to stop feeling so helpless. When you have an enemy you can see it, hear it or at least know what you are fighting up against. Alzheimer's is like the invisible enemy or sadistic monster. You know it is there consuming the one thing you love so much but you can't see it on an X-ray, or feel it, or even prove your loved one has it. There is no viable proof that Alzheimer's is consuming your loved one without an autopsy and then what difference does the "proof" make? Each day it takes another bite out of the one you love and then you are left with the leftovers of someone you don't even recognize anymore.

My mom was tough as nails. I rarely saw her cry. I have many old newspaper clippings indicating how she broke up a crime ring, or did this or that at the DPD. She never took any crap off me, ever. Yet, this disease was slowly, stealing her from me and everyone else.

I met so many people in the almost three years she was in Memory Care. Many of these had been in the law enforcement field, medical field, schoolteachers, lawyers, homemakers, a famous female pro golfer; the list goes on and on. At times the light would go off in the Alzheimer's patient's heads and the things they would say or share were remarkable, hilarious, thought inspiring and memorable. These were not ordinary people. I never met an Alzheimer sufferer who was ordinary, never.
Some patients were so clever, even in their disease. They could charm you into think- ing they were a nurse or a visitor. I was fooled a couple of times. If anyone ever thinks Alzheimer's is found in dumb people, let me assure you, it is not.

I truly believe my mom could have survived an atomic bomb. She would have been the one gathering food and water. She would have been the one keeping control while others were in shock. She would have been the one sewing, and mending clothes for everyone, or even cooking some of her favorite foods we all loved. She never would have been the one afraid or in need of taking care of.

She did not survive Alzheimer's.

The majority of those we met at the center when Mom first entered are all gone now. I watched many pass on while she was there. It broke my heart each time. There were those times towards the very end that I wished it had been her. They were free. They were not locked up inside the disease anymore. I knew how much my mom would have hated what she had become.

I still have no answers as to why some suffer longer than others. My Uncle, on my dad's side, died two days ago from Alzheimer's and he was in Memory Care less than a year. I explained to my dad that this was a true blessing.

Yes, my beautiful strong mother fought the good battle, and she did a damn good job. I miss HER; I don't miss what she became. And I forgive myself for having that feeling.

I miss her every day, but when I think of her, I see her as I did when I was a child or adult, before the disease when she was so healthy. I try not to think of the days when, or after, she faded away. I took care of that person. I loved that person because I was respecting my mother and the body she had once inhabited.

What a survivor she was!

Sh*t Happens In The World Of Alzheimer's

Alzheimer's is not a pretty realm to live in. People change in all areas. The brain begins to malfunction. I think of it as going backwards. The tapes in the brain start having 'glitches,' they start skipping. Some parts get scratched so badly they can never be replaced. The sufferer begins doing things that make you say things like, "My mother could never do that," or, "My mother could never say that." My mother slapped who, when, where, how!?" I watched her put corn in her tea one day a piece at a time. Slowly, methodically and not one piece went into her mouth. I have listened to her tell me how her father came and visited her. He has been dead over forty years.

I have changed her diaper, I have smelled her urine and I have cleaned her soiled pants.

One day I walked in her room and she had defecated in her trashcan. I have walked in her room while she was in the restroom and she asked me to help her defecate. She had forgotten how.

I have had to beg her to let me clean her dentures because the food was so caked on them it was disgusting.

I have wiped her nose, I have wiped her butt and I have bathed my own mother many times after she either had an accident, or got her dinner all over herself.

These are the times you put on a pair of gloves, stick your hand where it needs to go and pretend you are in another place and just do what needs to be done. The times I washed her dentures I pretended they were jewels. When I would put them back in her mouth I would tell her how beautiful she was and she would smile. It was all I needed to be repaid for what I had just done.

I remember telling my daughter one day about cleaning up after one of her bathroom mishaps and my daughter said, "I could never do that." I said, "Yes you could." We all can when it comes to love. We can and we would and we do!

The only thing that bothered me about any of this is that I just did not want my mom to know what I had to do for her. She would have been mortified. It would have upset her far more that it did me. I never wanted her to lose any respect she had coming to her. She was always so incredibly independent. I have to thank Alzheimer's for one thing. She never knew what was happening to her. Thank You God for small blessings.

Dancing with Mom

In my blog on Facebook. I shared the day Mom and I danced. In my adult life I had never danced with my mother. I am sure as I child I did, but I do not remember doing so. The day we danced was less than a year before I lost her. At this stage she was in her wheelchair most of the time. She was losing the ability to walk due to 'forgetting' how, and also pain she was having. On this day, music was playing in the "social" room and she stood up with some of her friends. They were pretending to dance by using their arms and hands. I felt compelled to dance with her. A friend was with me, and he videotaped it. As I look back now I see there were NO mistakes in our time together. God orchestrated every picture that was taken, every video, every conversation, every anything, for me to have now. It is like being in a helicopter and flying over a parade. God sees the whole production while you are just a participant in your own parade. He sees the beginning and the end. Thank you God, for the dance with my mom. It was just another time we connected and found each other again, one more memory I will cherish. Xoxo

We connected as we danced

She sat in her wheel chair looking around the room
The music slowly began to play
Some stood and two held hands
I watched as she sadly looked away
Where is she? I ask myself –
Why can't she wake up and be herself just once more?
I would settle for just one day, an hour, a minute or two
Just so I could ask her ... How can I help you?
What can I do?
It's as if I was compelled to walk over to her chair
And say...
Momma, let's dance. You be Ginger Rogers, I'll be Fred Estaire.
For just a moment we "perfectly connected".
I saw it in her beautiful eyes.

We danced a few steps; she looked at me and smiled
Then as quick as she had been with me, she was gone.
But, I was not sad. We had connected that day, and
I had danced with my mom.

Caregivers In The Realm Of Alzheimer's

Caregivers and caregiving are not always labeled as such. They can be neighbors, friends, police officers, court investigators, paralegals, attorneys, pastors, postal workers, counselors and sometimes complete strangers. God places who, and what, you need in your life right when you need them. This was one of the many lessons my mom's disease taught us.

I was so fortunate to have found some awesome people to help me with my mother. After getting some control of the abuse she suffered and obtaining guardianship of her, I was able to hire caregivers to come into her home. I hit the jackpot on two women who had their own company. The reason for starting their caregiving company was because their own mother had suffered with Alzheimer's.

We are all like family when we have an Alzheimer's sufferer amongst us. We know what we know without saying a word. We have been there and done that.

Patsy and Barbara owned Clear Choice Senior Care. I can honestly say I truly believe they were able to rescue my mom. Due to their care, I had more time with her I would not have had otherwise. After I was awarded guardianship, I could control how her pills were given and make sure she was fed properly every day. This also kept any outside influence affecting her and we were able to start picking her up and spending time with her again. The caregivers loved my mom and vice versa. They began taking her to church again and re-acclimating her to society. This was very good for her. We started making beauty shop appointments and monthly doctor's office visits. It had been so long since she had been properly cared for.

This was the first time in years I honestly felt some peace for myself and for my mom. Sometimes we asked Patsy from Clear Choice Senior Care if the caregivers could stay the night. They often did. When Mom was hospitalized once, they even stayed with her and helped us out. Clear Choice had the best service and we became personal friends. Patsy attended Mom's funeral and we still speak. I will always recommend my friend's loved ones who are ill to their care.

When your Alzheimer's sufferer begins to become more than you can handle, this is a decision you will need to make. You cannot let someone else make this for you. Also, don't let guilt be your guide. If you think you have to be the only one providing care for your loved one, you will be doing a real disservice to yourself and your loved one. If you become so tired and so frazzled that you become ill, which often happens to the caregiver, then you are more of a detriment to your loved one than an asset. Don't be a loving martyr and I mean that in the most loving way. Give yourself a break and get yourself some help. If you think you cannot afford it. I promise you, you cannot afford not to get some help, even if it is only one day a week. A few hours of rest is better than no rest at all. Your sufferer needs a break from you and you need a break from your sufferer. You will both be the better for it. Speak to those who understand what you are going through. You cannot be all and everything. It is not normal and it is not healthy. You can be there some of the time, or most of the time, but not all of the time.

I use to beat myself up because I did not try and get guardianship of my mom sooner. In my gut I knew things were not right with my mom and her care. I felt like she was not getting her prescribed medications. I felt like she was pulling away from the family. I knew she was very ill and not herself. She was rude and she was doing things she had never done before. She even changed her last name, which she was adamant that she would never do. She had been a Katzen for over 26 years. She had a legal forms stating she would remain Rosemary Katzen, and yet she had changed her name. My gut told me this was not normal. She was pulling away from me and from her own grandchildren. She was disagreeing with family she had been around all of her life. This clearly was not my mother in her right mind.

Obie Ezechi

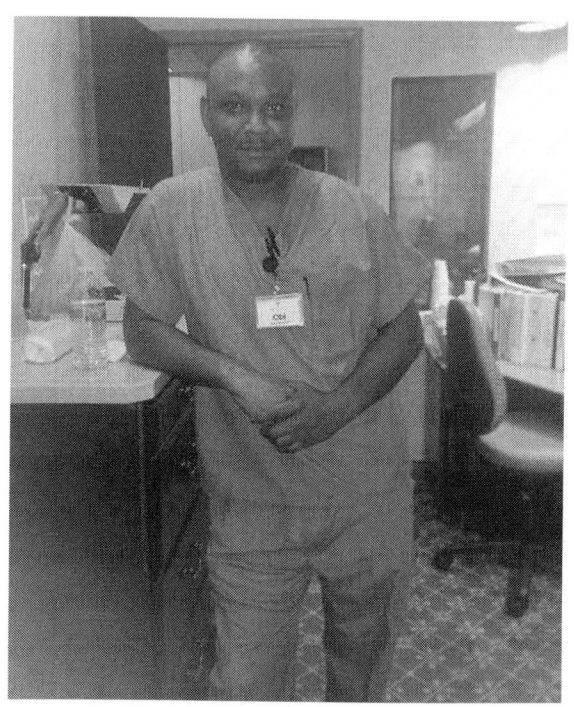

The first time I met Obie I was drawn to him. He was kind and had a warm demeanor. His smile was caring and contagious. I knew from his accent he was from Nigeria. Later, I found out he was from Enugu State in South Eastern Nigeria. He had been with the Memory Care Unit for two years when I met him. The first day we admitted Mom I was a basket case. I wanted to keep her at her home, but the courts were in charge even though I had guardianship, and their recommendation was for a Center. I looked long and hard to find the one where we placed her. Obie knew I did not want to leave her and he came and spoke to me. He was the nurse in charge at the unit. I cried for hours that first day and he assured me Mom would be well taken care of. He was in the unit with the more advanced stages of Alzheimer's sufferers. Mom would not go to his unit until a year later. I was actually happy when she was transferred, because then I knew that she was in the best hands possible. She was with her prince, since he called her his princess. Obie was patient with my mom even on those days that she was very ugly to him and to others. He explained to me, as I would apologize for her, that this was normal behavior. When she digressed and fought with others at the unit, Obie was the one to explain to me this was part and parcel of the disease, a stage they go through. No physician had passed this information on to me, but Obie did. He would text me when Mom had a special need. Those times that other helpers at the unit called and made me think the worst, Obie would calm my fears. He was not only a lifeline for my mother, he was the lifeline to my sanity at times. I soon found out he also worked with other Alzheimer's sufferers on a part time basis. This man was in the right position. The position of caring for those who could not care for themselves and he did not care what happened in the process to him, be it vomit, urine, blood or anything else. He was truly a great nurse with a huge heart. As I said, God assigned to me, and to Mom, exactly who we needed along our journey. Thank you to Obie and to the other workers who are there when we cannot be. To truly care for an Alzheimer's sufferer, I believe God must lead them, because it takes special people to care for someone who cannot care for themselves. We the family, depend on you to love and nurture those who mean *the absolute world to us*. Obie loved and nurtured my mom from day one. To this day, he still contacts me to see how I am doing. Obie, what a blessing you are to your profession. God bless you.

A Rose By Any Other Name…
Is Still A Rose

Alzheimer's disease is the most common form of dementia in those over the age of 65. As many as 5 million Americans age 65 and over may have AD, and that number is expected to double for every year interval beyond the age of 65. But Alzheimer's is only one of many dementia disorders; an estimated 20 to 40 percent of people with dementia have some other form of the disorder.

The dictionary defines it as a progressive mental deterioration that can occur in middle or old age, due to generalized degeneration of the brain.

The Mayo clinic definition states on the web, "Alzheimer's disease is a progressive disease that destroys memory and other important mental functions. It's the most common cause of dementia- a group of brain disorders that results in the loss of intellectual and social skills."

The above are medical examples of Alzheimer's. When you are experiencing your own loved one's symptoms, you may see all, some, or only a few of what are described above. You will have your own unique story to tell. We know our loved ones better than any doctor, therapist, or caregiver out there. We know their likes, dislikes and behaviors. Go by your gut. If it says to you that something is not right, listen and observe. Start taking action immediately. Spend more time watching your loved one. Write down those unique things they say that are abnormal. My mom began saying, occasionally, that she needed to retire. She had retired twenty years earlier when making this statement. She became increasingly more pessimistic about life. She trusted her family less and less, this was not my mother. I remember thinking; *she acts like she hates me.*

I took this on a personal level. I wish so many times I could go back and change this one specific aspect. It was not her; she definitely did not hate me. This was the disease eating up her brain. She pushed me away and until I realized she was sick and not just angry, I stayed away.

If your loved one "changes" in ways that are foreign to you, you don't have to run to the doctor right away. But, if the changes don't get better and you notice that you keep asking yourself, *why are they acting like this, this is just not them,* then maybe there is a problem.

There is no specific blood test for Alzheimer's. No x-ray that shows Alzheimer's as a specific diagnosis.

When going to a doctor. Your best bet is to see a Neurologist. There are Neuro Psychologist and Geriatric Psychiatrists. Remember, these are just my opinions. These doctors deal with the brain, and there are tests that can be given to rule out other factors that can possibly imitate Alzheimer's. These tests rule out the possibility of tumors and strokes

Alz.org states there is no single test that proves a person has Alzheimer's. A diagnosis is made through a complete assessment that considers all possible causes

*Medical History
*Physical Exam
*Neurological Exam
*Mental status tests
*Brain imaging

Some of these tests take hours. In the beginning I did not tell my mom I thought she had Alzheimer's. The reason being, I knew nothing about it. I thought maybe she had a stroke or some type of mental illness rearing its ugly head. She had been repeating herself and forgetting things. She knew through my years of nursing I was familiar with some doctors in the area and could find her a reputable one. She had spoken to me about her fears and I was ready and willing to help her in any way I could. I took her to her first doctor's appointment and many more in the years to come.

What You Will Need The Day You Place Your Loved One In Memory Care

First, take someone with you. A best friend, a member of the family. Someone you can lean on, someone to cry on their shoulder, because you will need it.

• Bring as many medical records as you can find.
• Bring their medicines in the bottles
• Social Security card
• Medicare card
• Special dietary instructions you may have
• Secondary insurance information
• Depends
• Plastic gloves
• Kleenex
• Tooth brush/tooth paste
• Sheets, pillowcases
• Clothing, pajamas, and comfortable shoes. Also socks without a slippery bottom. Elderly people are always cold. Make sure they have a nice warm sweater.
• Label ALL clothing. Put their name and the number of their room. Use a black marker.
• Leave all the jewelry at home. This may be hard for you if it is your spouse. It will be

worse if the jewelry comes up missing.

- Buy costume jewelry to replace the valued jewelry. They will not notice. Tell them you want to clean their jewelry and at that time replace it. Everything gets lost in these centers.
- I always took my mom some cream for her hands and feet. I loved putting cream on her. Alzheimer sufferers love touch and being touched. They can relate to this so much.
- The gloves are for you and the caregiver. Get them you will not be sorry.

Once they are in their room make it as homey as you can. They will need their own TV and bring pictures of everyone they know. Make a collage of those they love and place it on the wall so that when they wake up they see familiar faces. Put up pictures from home; use the same bedspread they use at home. Cover the mattress with a plastic mattress cover. They will have accidents. Take them a stuffed animal of some kind. It will comfort them. Do this for men also. Imagine you are moving their room and their belongings just to another locality. Keep everything as recognizable as possible. This will cause less stress. Always tell them you will be back soon, they are safe, you will take care of them. You love them and you are there for them, always, always, always.

Letter From Aunt Dot

I was in Mom's room and noticed she had a folded letter under some of her pajamas. It was folded into a tiny, small square. I opened it to find a letter. It started out telling someone how much they were missed and what was going on in their life. An old fashion type of letter someone would write a family member. I realized Mom had saved this. It did not belong to her, but with Alzheimer's she may think it did. There is no way to tell how it had gotten into her room. The same goes for the shoes under her bed that are not her size, and the three blouses that hang in her closet that are two sizes too small. Many of her own clothes are missing. I had longed given up on worrying about these things. In the world of Alzheimer's nothing really belongs to you, or maybe everything belongs to you.

After I read the letter it made me think of my Aunt Dorothy, who is my mom's last living sibling. She is three years older than Mom. I was closer to her than any of Mom's other sisters. Although she and Mom fought like cats and dogs, I know they loved each other. My Aunt Dot wrote Mom often. I could always expect a birthday card and also a Christmas card from her. Aunt Dot is one of those dinosaurs that still hand writes her letters and in the end she always talks about her faith and how God will bless you in some way.

This gave me a great idea. If Mom was saving someone else's letter then I knew she would want a letter from her own sister. I called my aunt up and explained all this to her. She was a little overwhelmed with Mom's illness. We all were. Aunt Dot adored Mom and did not know how to accept her illness. Mom was always the strong one, the tough broad who had it all together. She did not make mistakes. She did not get sick. She did not marry the wrong people and she most assuredly did not get a disease called Alzheimer's. My Aunt kept asking me over and over, "why" to all these questions. I had no answer.

My Aunt asked me what she should say in the letter. I explained to her to talk to Mom as if their parents were still alive, because Mom believed they were. I told her about 'love lies,' and to talk about the sisters and brothers, growing up, and so on. She seemed a little uneasy but said she would do it for Mom.

I was visiting Mom about ten days later. On her nightstand I noticed an envelope and it was from my Aunt Dot. I looked everywhere for the letter that should be enclosed. I could not find it. I started thinking that maybe Mom had thrown it away. Maybe I was wrong, maybe Mom did not want a letter from her sister. I continued to clean her room. Mom always hid things from herself. In her mind she was hiding them so she would not forget where they were, but of course she did forget. She had a drawer in her nightstand I used to find many things she would "hide." I found a knife for cutting food there, I found a stuffed animal Kenady had given her, I found scissors NO one had given her, I found a picture of myself, her and Mindy, and I also found Aunt Dot's letter folded into a small square. It was the same paper Aunt Dot always used. Lined paper torn from some notebook with the edges ripped out so as to almost look like lace with the holes still half way closed on the right side. Yes, that was her signature stationary. I loved it. Inside this paper treasure were the words of a sister who truly missed her sister. It told her how much she had wanted to visit, how often she thought of her and how many times she had wanted to call and speak with her. She then began to go over almost everything I had asked her to write. She brought up all the brothers and sisters, one by one. She talked about "Daddy," and the farm, and how they tended to the farm, and she brought up "Mom." She talked about school, how they played sports, and how they walked to school together. She spoke many times about their faith and attending church every time the doors were open. My Aunt Dot remembered everything verbatim I had asked her to talk about. I am sure this letter had triggered some memories in my mom's mind. It had to have.

At one point I thought about taking the letter home. I could use it in my book one day. I would even put it in there. As I started to refold it I heard a voice in my head that said, "Leave it." I always listen to what I believe is the voice of God. I placed it back into Mom's hiding place.

I never saw the letter again. I do see it often in my head. I often see my mom sitting on her bed or sitting in her chair reading it. Maybe she only read it once, maybe more. I know it must have meant something to her or she would not have hidden it. My mom was not the type of person to cry outwardly, fuss over someone, or show pain of any type. She had learned to keep most emotions inside. No matter what the letter from Aunt Dot had meant to her, she never would have said, even if she had been well. However, she would have taken the time to read it, fold it eight times and then put it in a special place.

I have a feeling Aunt Dot's letter is still out there. Maybe it is making its rounds. There could be different Alzheimer's sufferers finding the folded letter and reading it. I am sure it is, to this day, still making someone feel loved and cared for. We all need that, especially those who suffer with Alzheimer's.

Thank you, to my Aunt Dorothy Lee who has always taken the time to write to anyone who needed some love. She always has a kind word and a scripture or two. I think in my family there are many writers. We just have a different way of conveying our writing talent. My sweet, and loving Aunt Dot does it through her letter writing.

The Alzheimer sufferer speaks

The letter read so sweetly...

We miss you, we wish you were here
As I read it, I felt I was practically there
It made me feel good I could be anywhere
I did not feel so insecure, or so scared.

Hospice Care

I was going to make this one of my last chapters in the book, thinking it might be a subject people were most likely going to need help coping with. This one is a biggie. It goes to the core of your feelings.

While eating dinner tonight with a friend and after spending the weekend with my dad; I was feeling tired, but happy and content. It had been a great Thanksgiving. It was the first one without my mom. The first one I did not have to break up my time between the center, her, my daughter and the guilt that always came with holidays. The three questions I always asked myself were; should I try and get her to come home? Will she be sad if I don't try and get her home for the holidays? If by some miracle she did want to leave the safety of what she knew and go home, how would I take care of her needs and her fears?

Every holiday I asked myself these same questions. They would ruminate in my mind over and over again. This was the first Thanksgiving in years I could just wake up, get ready and go to my daughters. It had been a great day. A day with family. My dad being with me somehow took up the empty space that Mom had once occupied.

Now it is dinnertime on the day after Thanksgiving and I get a call from my Aunt. She tells me my Uncle, my dad's brother whom is also suffering with Alzheimer's, is in dire shape and they are calling Hospice. I can tell my Aunt is upset so I offered to call my dad. He was back in Oklahoma and I had time to think about what I would say to him.

Hospice was a godsend to us in our time of need. We chose Hospice Plus. Every one of those women I came in contact with were a gift from God. Hospice came in and took the "monkey" off my back so to speak. The one part of the Alzheimer's monster that hangs on long after you know in your gut that it is time for your loved one to go. The time when "they" are no longer there. Each time I saw my mother or this shell of who she used to be, I felt so sorry for her. It was as though she was speaking to me without speaking. She no longer had control of her bodily functions, could barely hold a cup to drink out of. She was given medicine to induce her appetite, could no longer walk, only whispered, rarely smiled and hardly ever did I hear that loud, contagious laugh. I would drive home after seeing her and ask God, "How much more? How much longer? How much more does she have to lose before she has lost everything?" I even prayed for God to take her home. Of course afterwards I felt such guilt. I wanted her to have freedom but mainly I wanted her to have her life back. This was no life, not for a woman like my mom. Alzheimer's had won. I was ready to admit defeat to the disease, but Mom and I had won the fight of our lives. We had bonded these last few years. We had the time we needed. We had the time to touch other's lives and we had the time to be a daughter and a mother, plain and simple. I had shared with her that I would one day write a book about her, and she had smiled. I would keep my promise.

So, when I got the call from my Aunt and I had to call my dad, I was actually content for him. My Uncle had been diagnosed about a year ago. My mom suffered for many years. I was happy for my Uncle that he would not have to suffer as long as Mom did.

When I made that call. I brought up the length of time I had to take care of Mom. I reminded Dad how hard it had been on her and on all of the family. My dad agreed. I then explained to him how his beloved brother, whom he called "Podnuh" for years, was now in the care of Hospice. Unexpectedly, my dad said he was ok with it because he knew it was best for his brother. He knew he would see him again one day. I felt a peace for my dad. I felt a peace for my uncle. He was now in the hands of angels here on Earth. Hospice was that to me. They walked into Mom's life and mine a few months before I lost her. They saved her from being force fed, and they went completely by her written wishes.

They were and are awesome. On Monday of this week I received a follow up letter from Hospice Plus. It has been less than a year now since I lost my mom. They sent me a letter that could help me with the first holidays without her.

I would recommend all those who are terminally ill to seek out a caring, loving and giving organization like Hospice. They are in your area. Ask your friends who may have used one. Get a good referral. Always, always, always keep good records. Make copies. Every organization will need your records. Do not expect professionals to keep records for you. Keep your own records. Stay up to date on their medications. Make multiple copies. When at the doctor's office, keep your receipts. Your receipts have diagnosis, dates and a wealth of information. The more information you have, the quicker, and easier, you will be able to get help for your loved one.

Last but not least, when it is suggested Hospice be called this does not mean your loved one is dying. My mom seemed to be on deaths doorstep until Hospice was called in. Many times our loved ones are overmedicated. Hospice will remove many of these meds if they are not needed. Mom was on two types of Alzheimer's meds. At that stage the meds were not making any difference and were actually making her less responsive. Let Hospice take over and trust them. This is their purpose. Their goal. They will do everything possible to give your loved one the care and dignity they deserve. Take a deep breath and throw that Alzheimer's monkey monster off your shoulders. You don't have to carry that burden anymore. Trust that God is going to take care of things. Believe it even if you really don't. Fake it, till you are there.

If you have a computer, go to your search engine and type in "Hospice." Many locations will come up. Call them. Speak to different agencies. If your loved one is in Memory Care they will also have recommendations. Have all your information in front of you when calling. Trust me, you will be emotional, and you won't remember or know by heart the answers to the questions you are asked. Have your folder and label it…"Alzheimer's and Mom or Alzheimer's and Dad or whomever. Have it with you always.

You will know when you have found the right Hospice care, God will guide you.

There Are Many Of Us And We Are Not Alone

When my dad got Alzheimer's disease, it was not specifically diagnosed nor was it clearly identified. The doctor was regularly doing memory tests, math quizzes and having him interpret abstract drawings.

However, the dementia progressed and it became clear to me that he had Alzheimer's. It is a very painful thing to see this in a parent. A parent who had always been funny, intelligent, engaging and loving.

I was told not to ask him, "Do you remember...?" but instead to say, "I remember when..." this is recommended, even if talking to someone else in the room. It is said to be comforting to the Alzheimer's sufferer.

My dad was a musician, so he was still able to play the piano, even as the disease progressed. Even in his last few weeks, he enjoyed a good back rub.

The piano playing, the back rubbing and the "I remember..." conversations helped me, probably more than him. It helped me to remember the "good old days" and to accept that this very distant man was, indeed, still my Dad.
-John

I had just graduated from nursing school when I noticed my father was acting different. He stopped fixing himself anything to eat, he would not get out of his chair, and he neglected to shave. He was always a clean, neat freak. This change in his personality came on so quickly we were not sure what was happening to him. The doctors have never completely said he has dementia or Alzheimer's, but they started giving him Alzheimer's medications to abate his condition. I would go to the store and buy him his groceries and would cry all the way there. I was unsure what to do about him. It has been 2 years now and he is still the same way. He has short term memory loss and asks questions over and over. I am the sole caretaker of him and I plan his every meal. He was a very independent father and always working, playing his hobby, or taking care of the house. He is very sweet to me and always tells me he loves me. When I was growing up this was not something he said. I told him that I wish he had told me that when I was young, and that maybe he didn't love me then. His reply was, "Well, time changes everything."

-Buffy

A HORRIBLY BEAUTIFUL JOURNEY

When I was asked to write of the horribly beautiful journey that was ours, from the day we once again heard the word "cancer" after so many years of living free from its shadow until now, I was hesitant to travel that road again. Some journeys leave a traveler forever changed no matter how many times the road is travelled.

My husband, Barry, developed Non-Hodgkin's lymphoma in 1994 when our son, Collin, was four months old. Following a stem-cell transplant from his brother, he had been cancer-free for seventeen years but had dealt with numerous side effects, including sensitivity in the lining of his cheeks. Because it was a familiar problem, I didn't pay much attention at first when I passed the bathroom door one day in August 2011 and caught sight of Barry swabbing the inside of his mouth. Meeting my eyes in the mirror, he said that there was something in his mouth that wasn't quite right. With that ordinary statement began a five month journey through a landscape that was familiar yet frighteningly new. This included doctor visits, tests, surgeries, and difficult decisions. We had been there before, but thankfully, just as before, we drew closer together instead of growing apart. God's presence, our love for each other as a family, and Barry's eternal optimism were our beacons in the dark. Our travel companions along the way were, at times, comforting and welcomed. Our friends offered hugs, cards and words of encouragement that were received at unexpected times, and practical offerings that were actually precious gifts. We learned that food given in love feeds both the soul and the body, and that having someone offer to do the dishes when you're too tired to think, is a treasure beyond price.

However, sometimes in our journey's darker places, we had other companions who were not so welcomed but had to be endured, they were panic, fear, depression, doubt. I must admit, those companions were usually invited along by me. Ironically, the person the world viewed as ill and weak was everyone's rock and the strongest of us all. Barry's doctors and nurses, many of whom became friends along the way, were amazed and touched by his sense of humor and indomitable spirit in the face of his rapidly worsening state. Years before, Barry had been chosen to be an Olympic torch-bearer due to his unstoppable determination, but I believe the greatest testament came from the surgeon who worked tirelessly to remove the tumor in Barry's mouth, and reconstruct his face and throat afterward. When Barry passed away in January 2012, I received a note from the surgeon, saying that he had never met a man like Barry and he had no doubt that, through knowing him, he himself had become a better doctor and a better man. This was amazing coming from a man who, initially, had such a bad bed-side manner that I was tempted to knock him through a wall! Barry's sense of humor stopped me from doing that, by the way. After the doctor said a particularly infuriating thing in the exam room upon our first meeting, Barry could feel me bristling. As I opened my mouth to engulf the doctor in a stream of choice words, I saw Barry behind the doctor's back, making a cross with his fingers, his eyes twinkling but begging me to behave. To this day, I'm sure the doctor wonders what made me burst out laughing in the middle of a serious consultation!

I learned so many beautiful lessons from Barry in the midst of our journey together. From him, I truly learned how to live and how to die. First and foremost, I witnessed that peace and joy are not tied to outward circumstances, and that love truly is the greatest gift of all. One day, after witnessing a married couple who obviously were having problems, Barry hugged me close and asked, "Aren't you glad that all we have to deal with is a little disease?" Toward the end, when Barry was still optimistic but I knew there would be no healing for him in this world, the knowledge that love is eternal is what sustained me. I don't know how people who have no faith deal with death. The belief that this world is all there is would make death unbearable for me. After Barry's passing, it helped me so much to picture Barry as once again healthy, whole and waiting for me until we can be together once more. In the meantime, as I work to build a new normal without him, I am strengthened by memories of love, joy and incredibly gentle power.

I began my story by calling my journey "horribly beautiful," but it is so true that beautiful lessons come out of adversity. In the first weeks after Barry's diagnosis, I received a poem that sustained me then and continues to do so to this day...

The Oak Tree

A mighty wind blew night and day.

It stole the oak tree's leaves away,
Then snapped its boughs and pulled its bark
Until the oak was tired and stark.
But still the oak tree held its ground
While other trees fell all around.
The weary wind gave up and spoke,
"How can you still be standing, Oak?"

The oak tree said, "I know that you
Can break each branch of mine in two,
Carry every leaf away,
Shake my limbs, and make me sway.
But I have roots stretched in the earth,
Growing stronger since my birth.
You'll never touch them, for you see,
They are the deepest part of me.
Until today, I wasn't sure
Of just how much I could endure.
But now I've found, with thanks to you.
I'm stronger than I ever knew."
-Johnny Ray Ryder, Jr.

Here's to true strength. Thank you, Barry for helping me know what it looks like. I love you, now and forever.
-Karen Corkern -

The Mother of a Honky Tonk Angel

Sometime around January of 2000, my Mother was diagnosed with dementia. She was 75 years old so this came as no surprise. I knew what this meant, she would start to forget a few things, and ask the same question over and over. No big deal. Otherwise, her health was really good for her age.

Fast forward to 2003, when she was diagnosed with full on Alzheimer's. I knew the basics and knew this is one of the most awful diseases out there. It robs the patient of their mind and most of all their dignity. It is a tireless disease. My Mom hardly ever went to sleep, which meant someone had to watch her 24/7. We were able to have hospice come in and check on Mom, but they constantly recommended we put her in a "facility" to deal with her condition. This was out of the question.

In 2005, Mom suffered a minor stroke, and the Doctor wanted her to go to rehab to build up her strength. At least that is the story we told her. It was, in fact, one of those "facilities." Somewhere in her brain she recognized this facility for what it was, and quickly became a person to be watched. She was given a really nice ankle bracelet which sounded alarms if she attempted to leave the facility. Mom broke out of this Facility three times and went un-noticed. The third time, I was in my car going to see her and at the busiest intersection in North Plano, stood my mom. I had to do a double take. At first, I thought what on earth is that poor woman doing with no shoes on, in the middle of the street? Then it dawned on me that it was Mom. I think I had an out of body experience. I stopped traffic, picked her up, and got her in my car. I attempted to go to the facility to let them know I had just found her, when she began to cry and beg me not to take her back. I told her I was going to pick up her belongings.

I took Mom home and got a nice bubble bath ready for her. It was then that I noticed all the awful bruising she had, especially in between her thighs. I became upset but tried to maintain a normal behavior around her. I got her cleaned up, and called the police. I filed a formal complaint against the facility.

Mom and I had talked prior to her getting really sick with this disease, she wanted a graveside service, and she did not want to be embalmed. She had also told me what songs she wanted and which prayers. Mom wanted me to read her eulogy. What I did not know, was the funeral home will not touch a person who has not been embalmed. This meant in 2006, when Mom passed away, I went to the funeral home to wash her and put her clothes and make-up on her for the last time. Also, it had to be a closed casket. I have had people ask me, how you could do this? My answer is also, how could I not?

Her service was beautiful; she was taken to the graveside in a country wagon, drawn by two magnificent black horses. She arrived at the graveside greeted by one of her songs, "How Far is Heaven" by the Los Lonely Boys. I read her eulogy and prayers, we played another song, "Lord Loves a Drinking Man" by Kevin Fowler. It was everything she wanted.

-Anonymous

I was asked to write about what it is like being a Hospice nurse that works with patients who have Alzheimer's. In order to answer that question, I must back up a bit. I am somebody who never thought I would be a Hospice nurse. I have worked on a cancer floor, and for six years on a Medical and Surgical floor. I then worked in a rehabilitation facility for 3 ½ years. I routinely gave medications and carried out treatments and doctor orders. Being a Hospice nurse is different; you are trying to make the patient as comfortable as possible and to live out their last days as they wish.

Often when asked, "What do you do for a living?" I answer, "I am a hospice nurse." I prepare myself for what follows. Usually it is a wrinkled brow or a disapproving grimace. Then the conversation might go something like, "How do you do that?" Or, "Wow, you must be a strong person." I will then nod my head approvingly and say," I like what I do." I explain that I was brought to Hospice for a reason, but that's usually as far as the conversation will go. But, perhaps what I should say is, "No, I am not the strong one; it is the patient's loved ones who are the strong ones." This is especially true for the family of an Alzheimer's patient. All disease is terrible and nondiscriminatory, but Alzheimer's is the very cancer infecting and affecting ones memories. We must not fool ourselves, because there is an epidemic of Alzheimer's in this country. The Alzheimer's patient is a mother, a father, a daughter, a son, a grandfather or a grandmother. Alzheimer's patients are nurses, firemen, police officers, war veterans, volunteers, and doctors even. Alzheimer's can happen to anyone.

As a hospice nurse, I am invited into these patient's lives and I am privileged to hear stories of my patient's lives before their diagnosis. Also, to be invited into their homes where I often see photos of happier times. I still cannot get over how everyone looks like a movie star on their wedding day.

My words are for the loved ones of a patient with Alzheimer's, who love long and hard and give all they have. To the loved ones who attempt to hold on and to never let go of the fading image of the person they know and love. They are the strong ones, not me. **-Katrina DeAnn Montenegro**

I was 30 years old when my Mom was diagnosed with Alzheimer's. There were noticeable difficulties with her memory and sense of direction. It wasn't diagnosed until she was in the hospital with terminal cancer. The results from a brain scan showed gray matter and what they believed to be Alzheimer's. Within months we went from having our regular conversations, to not having any conversation. The morphine only added to, and sped up, the decline. My world was turned upside down. I lost her even before she passed, which was shortly after. Fourteen years later my Dad was diagnosed with Dementia. Here I was dealing with this horribly awful disease again. Just a different form, or maybe just a different name for the same disease and the discomfort that affected all of us. While it is slower at progressing, and we've been able to have many wonderful conversations in spite of it, it has changed him. Part of him is gone, the dad I knew and loved is no longer here. I wondered if this was God's way of easing the transition of losing my parents. But, was I just trying to fool myself and hope this was God somehow trying to ease some of the pain I was feeling? God would not want to hurt me, would He? Of course not, I kept telling myself. I read an article that spoke of the chances of an adult child developing the same disease. The statistics are scary. Especially when it's both parents. I've never read another article or statistic since then. If I have to live through it as well, I'll do it when the time comes, not beforehand. I don't fear or hate Alzheimer's or Dementia. I feel I have to respect what my parents experienced throughout their journey here on earth. I will always miss those talks with my mom about whatever was going on in our lives, and that connection. She had a way of making me feel everything would turn out for the best. How unconditionally loved she made me feel. My Dad had a way of making me feel equally safe and loved. I will never forget their love for me. My mom still lives in me and many others comment on my caring nature. I truly believe this is my mom living on in and through me.

I just wanted to share that I met Mary on Facebook many years ago and followed her journey with her mom. I could relate to so many of her stories. We shared so many of the same catastrophic moments. All of us with parents who have Alzheimer's have a special bond. I am sure Mary and I will be friends forever. It was not Alzheimer's that brought us together, but the love we shared for those who suffer with it.
-Rose Bayer

Alzheimer's is a horrible disease, a friend of Warren's, my significant other, works in a care home and said that some of the patients in there had the most brilliant minds; a former pilot, teachers, nurses, scientist. Alzheimer's can affect anyone from a road sweeper to the most highly educated and academically clever people. No one is immune to this dreadful disease. I am dealing with it myself in my own life. Sometimes it just helps to have someone to talk to and bounce things off of; someone that is dealing with the same circumstances you are. At our worst times, we can at least depend on the fellowship of those just like us and in the same circumstances.
-Leonie Hyatt

Losing someone can be very tough, and I'm not very good at dealing with death. I don't even think anyone is to be honest. Rosemary (Nana) Katzen was a lady of honor, courage, and respect. She could always make you smile by just seeing her. I remember the nice days outside we used to have. Throwing a big bouncy ball in the yard, drinking lemonade, talking about what I learned in my pre-K class over the last week, eating hot dogs, and just having the most fun anyone could have. I loved her more than anything. Then I realized that something was different about her. "What is she doing?" I wondered. The days that I came to the house, she was always, I mean always, wearing makeup. But then she wasn't. That's odd, I thought to myself. Maybe she just didn't want to that day so, whatever. But then other things started happening. At one point she kept saying someone else's name, not mine. Maybe that was a mistake too. But weird things just kept happening day by day. Now I'm going to be honest, I don't remember this day, but my parents do. Back when Nana used to watch my sister and me, she was very careful and gentle with us. Now I remember this part clear as day. I was in the living room coloring a picture, then suddenly, I heard a sound. THUMP! Then I heard crying, it was Kenady. Nana had accidentally dropped her. We took her to the hospital, and it turned out, she was okay. She needed a couple of stitches, but other than that she was perfectly fine. After the incident happened, we didn't really go over there that much, unless we were with our parents. As I got older, I started to realize what was wrong with her. GG, my gorgeous grandma, had told me that she had a disease called Alzheimer's. It was when old people start to have trouble remembering things, and have loss of short term memory. I would say, about two years ago, the start of third grade, was the year that she moved into her new nursing home. Nana loved it, she'd always tell me what she did that day and how much fun she had. And if she was happy, I'm happy. About one year later in April I'd say, she was definitely different. I looked at my mom and I said, "She's different." Then my mom had told me that she was getting sick and it may be her time soon. A couple weeks later we went to her nursing home. I sat in the dining room with her while my parents were cleaning her room. I was talking to her about school, and my grades and then we stopped talking for a few minutes. And out of nowhere, Nana starts laughing. I was looking around to see what was so funny. Nothing there. So I asked her what was so funny. All she said to me was, "Shhhh." Then she just stopped, and I asked her one more time and said, "Nana, why were you laughing?" She said, "Well, I'm surprised you're not laughing, Murray just told the funniest joke I have ever heard." For a second I was puzzled. Who's Murray? I thought to myself. Then it clicked. Murray was Nana's first husband that had died five years before I was born, after a heart attack. I went and told my mom about it. She told GG and they talked about it. What could it mean? No one knew. She died five

weeks later. March 11, 2015. Like I already said, Nana was a lady of respect, honor, and courage. I will always love her and never, EVER, forget about her.
-Bradyn Stevens (great grandson to Rosemary Katzen)

You don't know what you can do until you are faced with doing it.

Dad lived with us for 5 years and I wouldn't change a thing except taking better care of ourselves. When you are caring for someone else it is easy to ignore your own needs. I did try working during the years that Dad was here, but being the chauffer, the cook, the laundress, the nurse, the homemaker and all around caretaker made it difficult to do a good job for both a company and my family.

My dad never wanted to go into assisted living and we did not want to put him there either. But in reality WE were his assistants. It was small things at the beginning, but as dad lost more and more of what he could manage, we stepped in to fill the gap. He constantly thanked us and said he could never do this on his own. Even though we had family that came into town from time to time to let us go on vacation, it wasn't enough time to nurture ourselves. We had pages of notes on Dad's medication, food preparation, directions to the center he went, directions to the hospital in case it was needed, directions to the doctors, bed time routine, and the list goes on. At times it was more stressful to leave than to stay. Friends and family say they understand, but they have no clue. That is not their fault, that's just how it is. They come and help for short periods of time and then go back to their lives. We didn't have much of a life anymore. The only time we both panicked was bringing Dad in home hospice care. It was over-whelming. We looked at each other and didn't know if we could do it or not. I spoke with my cousin Susan that day and she had told me how she went through hospice 3 times in one year with loved ones. It gave me the encouragement we needed. Hospice was wonderful! Ten minutes before dad passed on he was telling his hospice nurse joke after joke! He had an amazing life and loved to make people laugh! If I can go out as gracefully, it will be a blessing! Dad was surrounded by the people that loved him the most when he left this world!

If I could give one word of advice when being a caretaker it would be, don't forget yourself!! And if you know of a caretaker please don't forget about them. They need encouragement, breaks from the usual, or just a good shoulder to cry on! Being a caretaker is the biggest blessing and also the hardest. Helping a loved one leave this world with dignity is the greatest honor you can have.

-Jasper Manderachia September 14, 1921 –July 22, 2015
Marilou & Mike Castelli Official Caretakers

YOU ARE MY VOICE

You are my voice
When I cannot be heard
When I am sick
Or can't say a word

Please don't be quiet
But instead speak your mind
Make sure my caretakers
Are hardworking and kind

Please cry out for me
When my voice has been hushed
Make sure I'm clean and well dressed
And that my meals are not rushed

Please don't be silent
When I can't make a sound
You are my only chance
At not being silenced and bound

I cannot say
What I think or how I feel
This memory disease
Is simply unreal

Sometimes in the night
I want to shout and scream
This is not fair
Is it a nightmare or dream?

You are my voice
So please don't be still

I may not remember
But my heart still feels

-Kimmy
For Momma Mary
May 2015

Dr. Williamson is a professional and personal friend of mine. I worked for a Rheumatologist for many years and we shared an office with Orthopedic Associates. Dr. Williamson started this practice in the 70's and it has grown to include many physicians and now has two locations. I knew him professionally and was also a patient of his at one time. I was fortunate to be best friends with his nurse, Janice Boudreau. He has been an orthopedic surgeon since 1976, performing over eight thousand surgeries. On August 4th 2011, he suffered a massive stroke and his life has forever changed. I asked Dr. Williamson to give me his experience with physical loss versus neurological damage as in the case of Alzheimer's.

Words as written by **Richard W. Williamson**, M.D.

The thing that is very apparent to me is that there are two parts of the loss with Alzheimer's. The physical part I am much more familiar with. I was once an avid skier, and I can remember that first warm day of spring when the water is cool and the sun is shining. When you jump in and get goosebumps as you grab the rope, cut outside the wake and edge in toward the gate, picking up speed. Your cheeks are billowing out with the wind, and the spray is sticking to your legs. You may have to wrap your calf with duct tape to keep the skin from peeling back. Then you lose all of that, and you lose the ability and the sensation of speed, acceleration, exhilaration, and that is bad. But, there is something more important and that is the sensory side of things. Say I meet a beautiful woman. Am I going to be able to experience the smell, the touch, the taste, the softness of her skin, the warmth of her neck against my lips, her smile, the quick beating of my heart, the tightening in my groin, and the unmistakable sensation of being very attracted to someone? How much of that is going to be gone? How much will the sensations be dampened, the smell and taste be blunted, and the sensation be lost? It is easy for me to say. I have 60% of my proprioception and 60% of my sensation on the left side of my body, but there is so much more to life than just sensation and touch and proprioception, and anybody who has ever been in this situation knows what I am talking about. Although the physical is difficult to lose, especially when it is something you are proficient in, it is not nearly as big of a loss as the emotional and

*sensory side, which makes up the other part of the brain. I think it would be much easi-
er to live without the physical side of things than the emotional side of things, and I am
glad my brain is still intact, although my body is not. It gives me hope for the future far
beyond nearly losing the exhilaration of the physical side of life. So, there is a saying
that you can adopt and that is, "all you can do is all you can do." You work, you try to
get better, and you try to gain back independence, but in the meantime you don't shut
off your mind and you try to experience life.*

This is Dr. Williamson's experience with the physical loss due to stroke, versus the
neurological loss due to Alzheimer's. In the case of a stroke and paralysis, although the
thought is horrific if we allow ourselves to think of it, we would still have that "hope"
Hope comes from cognitive abilities and they would remain intact, even when our
physical abilities might be deteriorated. If the mind remains unbroken, and unimpaired
then we can still have hope.
Alzheimer's offers no hope or change for its sufferer, and without hope we lose that
thinking that what we wish or pray for … is attainable.

The Pool With A Heart

I had a dream one night that Mom's backyard had a pool in it. Was this Mom
telling me to put a pool in the yard? I knew this would be something she would approve
of, because it was an indulgence that would pay off. It would help me to keep a promise I had made to myself years ago.

As far back as I can remember I have waged a battle against weight. My mom
was always a perfect size eight, and I do mean perfect. Me, on the other hand, I was no
perfect size, period. I was not obese, but during my teenage years there was no such
thing as cute clothes for girls my size, or stores such as Torrid, Lane Bryant or Junior
large sizes. At most I was twenty pounds overweight, but over the years this became
a much bigger issue. After I was in a car wreck and broke my back, my weight sky-

rocketed. My mom always wished I was smaller. She was not the only one. In 2000 I started swimming and lost a lot of weight. By 2005 I was smaller than I had been in high school and my mom was very, very proud of me. In 2008 my mom paid for me to have a tummy tuck. I finally had a beautiful body and I was now smaller than she was. I don't know who was happier, Mom or me. I lost the weight primarily from swimming. I became an avid swimmer, swimming three days a week. I got so good at it; I could do a mile in 35 minutes. I did this without a break. The time she began to show signs of her illness, I was not as disciplined. She became my primary concern and my swimming became a lesser concern. I quit my job to take care of her and her needs.

While my mom was ill and in Memory Care in 2012, she would often comment on how pretty she thought I was and for me not to get fat again. We both laughed. I knew her desire for me to remain healthy would be one of the last things she would ever forget.

So, here I was carrying around an extra few pounds I had gained from not swimming due to my care giving. Was this dream something she had sent to me or was it from God? Either way, I spoke to Mindy and it had always been a dream of mine to have my own pool. I called Pool Stop and that is how I met Stephen Thompson. With the plan of the pool came the idea of burying some of Mom's favorite things at the deepest part of the pool. Steve showed up one day with a box he had made for me to put these things in. On the day they put the plaster in, he showed up with a heart made out of one of the tiles used on the inside of the pool. This went on top of the box already buried. Since the pool is very small, I had jets installed so I can swim against them. This pool is primarily for exercise, but I have gotten so much more from it. Each time I swim in the pool, I go down to the bottom and touch the heart. I never knew you could cry under water. Thank you, Harvey Rippy for a dream come true.

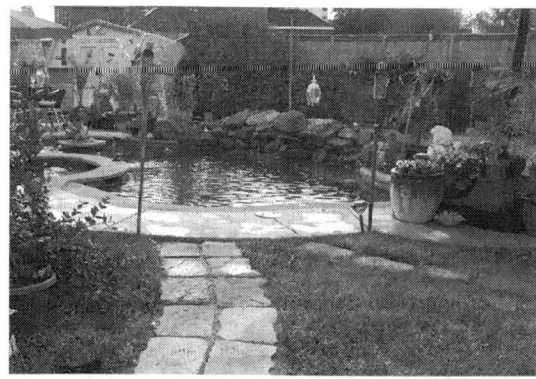
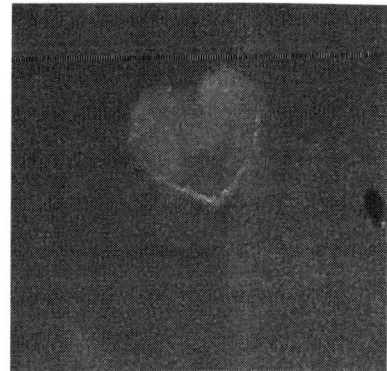

Let God Have Control, Take A Brief Pause For Rest

During my mother's last few years in her disease I was quite busy trying to control everything around her. If I had no control over the disease and what it was doing to her, then I would try even harder to control the other circumstances. I made sure her room smelled good, I made sure she always had sugar-free chocolate in her fridge that we put in her room, and I always bought her new pajamas. She spent so much time now in leisure clothes or just sleeping, and of course, the shoes had to match the clothes. If she was going to be a mess in her head, I would make sure physically she was not messy. I could tell mom was giving up. She had always worn dentures. She had the most beautiful smile, and she took a lot of pride in her "teeth" and God forbid anyone should know she wore dentures. This was a secret she told no one. If you did know, you would still never see her without her teeth. A few of the workers in Memory Care have said she took her teeth out occasionally. I had a hard time believing this. That was not my mom!

One day when I visited, she was eating her meal. I watched in horror as she removed her bottom dentures and began cleaning them at the dinner table in front of all the others. She was fine with it. I was aghast. I clearly explained to her that this was not appropriate. My God, who was I talking to? She clearly was gone, my mom anyway. This was one of those times that I knew in my gut there was little left of my mother.

The signs are all there. As I said, the loved one will know. We know before anyone else. Just like me, it took the dentures to bring me to reality. I had to stop fighting, I had to let go. No matter how many clothes and sugar-free chocolate I brought her, she was still going to die with this horrible disease. She began keeping her mouth closed when it was time to take her meds. I would get calls from frantic workers stating she was rude and refused her meds. At first, I would run up there and cajole her to take them. She usually got mad at me and yelled for ME to take the damn things. At first this drove me nuts. I would beg, make jokes, or call Obie. I would do anything I could think of to get her to take them. I didn't realize until later that this was her way of saying enough is enough. She was tired of this crap, of this life.

In the latter part of 2014 she was rarely eating and they put her on some medicine to induce her appetite. When she did eat, it was sporadically and she made strange combinations out of her food. Sometimes I had to look away. My inclination was to hand feed her and she seemed to like that. Other times she did not want any food. I stopped fighting her, I allowed her the freedom to just be, and let go.

The first part of 2015 she was really digressing and she was now with Hospice. Hospice Plus was a true gift from God. This is when I met Amanda Maxwell, Katrina Montenegro, and Debbie York. Katrina was the RN who I did all the paperwork with. We immediately became friends. Hospice took over, took her off most of the meds she was taking, except for the ones for her diabetic needs, and she honestly improved for a bit. She slept more than she was awake, but health wise she had improved. I cringed every day when I had to go and visit her. *How much worse could she get*, I asked myself? How much more dignity would be taken away from her? I wanted to fulfill the promise I made long ago. I explained to Katrina there were to be no heroes in Mom's case. If she was to die then by God let her go. I put the sign up in her room. I even told Obie, because of his kind heart. Do not bring her back to life if she has a heart attack. I was adamant about letting her die peacefully to get out of this hell that she now called her life and existence. I was adamant about getting guardianship to protect her from any evil. I would protect her in life and in her death. This was my mother. I would be damned if something worse happened and she was in some vegetative state and had to live like that. How could I live with myself if she had to live that way? They may have thought the "sweet Mary" had turned into some "mean bitch," but I was not here to fulfill any promise to them. I was here to fulfill a promise to her.

On March the 2nd Mom broke her hip. We never got the exact story. We never even received the incident report. It was something to the effect that she stood up out of her wheelchair, someone called her name, she turned to look at them and then she lost her balance. When the call came in I was in shock. Although Mom was very weak and damaged mentally from her disease, I still felt like she was a female version of the Hulk. She was still strong, and looked healthy from the neck down. When I would change her, I could still see the taught muscles in her legs, and the biceps in her arms. Up until the last few months she would still occasionally let out that big strong laugh of hers. I was the one having the hardest time with the change in my mother. The reason being, I knew her before, and what was left was a remnant of what she had been at one time.

When an Alzheimer's sufferer needs an operation after a fall such as Mom's, you will need to take time to make this decision. Do you really want to put them through something they will not understand, move them to yet another new place? When I got the call about Mom needing surgery for her broken hip all I could think of was, *how much more pain does she have to experience? How will this help with her quality of life?*

The call came from my daughter; Mom had fallen and broken her hip. Mindy had told them to take her to the hospital. I was livid at myself for missing the call. I called and got all of the information I could and then called the Emergency Room at hospital. I explained I had guardianship and wanted to speak with someone who could help me. I said, "Please understand my mom will not make any sense, she has Alzheimer's." They said they were so glad I had called. Mom was in a jovial mood and making everyone laugh. I explained I would come up there and they said I should wait until she had a room, I would really just be in the way. First thing in the morning I got many calls, a lot of advice stating she needed surgery. I felt like I was on a Ferris wheel and it had lost control. I was spinning faster and faster. Here I was left with the decision to operate on my mom. She would not understand, she would never recover, and there would be no physical therapy. She was with Hospice, she was dying. A nurse spoke with me and said Mom would be in pain if she did not have surgery. How could I say no? I prayed about it and Mindy and I decided on the surgery. I could not imagine her dealing with pain. I had no idea where we would go from here.

We saw her early before her surgery. She was very confused. She hardly spoke and acted as though she did not know either of us. I truly believe she gave up, she had laughed her last time, spoken her last words the night before. She was gone and I knew it in my gut. I was feeling guilty for putting her through the surgery. The doctor had expressed it was 50/50 chance she would make it through the surgery. She was having problems with her heart. Inside I was screaming at God, the same repeat question, *how much more do You want her go through?* I expressed to the doctor I wanted no heroics. He explained to me that due to their oath he would have to use every means possible to save her life, albeit her DNR. I was not happy with this decision and he even expressed he was not happy with having to make it.

Immediately after Moms fall we decided to put her in a home health care environment. No more memory care homes with so many people to look after. This would be my choice if I had it to do over. Many people are turning their houses into homes for live in care-giving. I find this much more personal for the sufferer and the family.

We found a home close to mine and it only had six Alzheimer's patients living in it. I was happy about our decision. We moved all of Mom's furniture and personal items there. When Mom came in I noticed her teeth were not in her mouth. I was so upset. Here I was again thinking Mom would, by some miracle, wake up, be normal and be screaming for her teeth. I had to get her dentures Hospice, and every person involved in Hospice, went out of their way to help me, including finding my mom's dentures. It was mind-boggling. This was another way God was showing me HE was in control. I could let go and let Him be in charge.

After the surgery, Mom was transferred to the new place. Even in this late stage, after surgery and knowing I was losing her; you still have that tiny ray of hope your loved one will miraculously be healed and walk away unscathed. I spoke to the surgeon later. I asked him what the plan was since she had late stage Alzheimer's. He seemed shocked and said the prognosis was not good, but the surgery would keep her from having undue pain. I asked if this was true then why did we put her through the surgery. He said if he had known she was in Hospice, he probably would not have done the surgery. At first I was angry. Then I decided it would not change her predicament and he did what any doctor would do if left in the dark. I think some people forget that Alzheimer's sufferers "feel" just like anyone does. They just don't have a voice anymore. I don't mean that they can't speak, they just have difficulty expressing. This is left to a loved one. I don't know whom else I could have told that Mom has Alzheimer's and is in Hospice Care. You think you dot all your " I's" and cross all your" T's," but sometimes you don't even feel heard yourself. So, at that time you move on to what can be done for her now. With an Alzheimer's loved one you can't think in terms of the future, you have to focus on the now, this moment.

I wish I could say Mom's stay at the individual home we found for her was a good one, but it was not. I felt I was not listened to, and her individual personal requests were not followed. She really never woke up at the home. Hospice was called in for 24-hour care. She no longer wore her dentures, did not open her eyes and rarely made any connection with any of us. She was dying and I knew it. Of course, I wanted to pick her up, sit her in a chair and cajole her into eating. But, this was not her wish. I stood next to her bed, talked to her and pretended she could hear me. I called all those I knew and clearly explained she was dying. I left to get her some meds she needed. When I returned she was positioned upwards in a chair being fed, force-fed in my opinion. I asked where her DNR was. It clearly explained she did not want to be fed if she was in this type of predicament. I was livid. I could tell she was uncomfortable. At first I just stood there and was silent. I had finally had enough and I said so. The nurse/ owner of facility finally stopped but left her sitting up in the chair. I could honestly FEEL my mom's pain. Her breathing seemed worse. The nurse left and I asked where the copy of DNR was. No one seemed to know. After it was found by a worker in the safe I took the paper and wrote on it. "I am the guardian of my mom...this DNR will be followed." I then wrote in big letters "THERE ARE TO BE NO HEROES... you will specifically go by the DNR she has signed." Katrina Montenegro came up to me and I was crying. She told me she understood and she would get 24 HR care for mom so she could pass in peace. Katrina was my Hero that day. I understand any person in the medical field wants to save a sick individual. But, I believe you should look at the facts, check with the family, the diagnosis, and then make an educated choice. No one has the right to go against another person's personal wishes. My mother's DNR stated specifically she never wanted to be force fed. That decision to stop feeding a parent or loved one is the hardest decision you will ever make. It is a decision of pure love and of "letting go."

My mom passed a few days later. Her way, her wishes, with dignity and re-spect for what she wanted. I had my time with her; the day God gave me the day before she died.

What I want to share about this experience is to go by your gut. If a "profes-sional" tells you a loved one needs to eat and they are dying, listen to the voice inside of you. Ask your family. Most of all do what your loved one wanted. If they took time to fill out a DNR, or were adamant about certain things, then we as the loved one need to respect what THEY wanted. It would be a dishonor to do otherwise. We can't do what we want and we must certainly cannot allow others to do what they feel is best for someone they do not know. Stand up for THEIR rights!

My most sage advice is to ask those you trust for their advice and then make your decision. Guess what? If you make the wrong one, it is ok. You are going through a lot, and have been through more than most. You deserve to make a less than perfect decision. Nothing is written in cement. It is a learning experience and believe it or not, most likely *it will be the right decision* in the end. God does not expect perfection from us. We need to accept we are making our decisions from a place of love, not from a place of professionalism. So, it will be the right decision. God is with you, just like He was with me. Relax as much as you can, pray and when you look back (just as I did) you will see how God was there the whole time. You will not be alone. All of us who go through this will be there with you in "spirit". We are a message away, a webpage apart, a phone call waiting. We understand.

1 Corinthians 13:4-7New International Version (NIV)
4 Love is patient, love is kind. It does not envy, it does not boast, it is not proud. 5 It does not dishonor others, it is not self-seeking, it is not easily angered, it keeps no record of wrongs. 6 Love does not delight in evil but rejoices with the truth. 7 It always protects, always trusts, always hopes, always perseveres.

While writing my dialogue on Facebook, which inevitably became the book "Fading Image," I was reminded numerous times how love entered into the equation. Many times I would think to myself; this is the most horrific thing I have ever gone through in my entire life, watching my mother slowly fade away before my eyes, yet God keeps showing me such love through others. Where does this abundance of love come from? How can I feel such patience for my mother's incessant repeated questions, or do such impossible things that would revolt me before? This is the love that does not boast, the love that does not anger. This was the same love that gave me the idea of asking her caregivers at the Memory Care unit what I could do to help them, to help her? The same love that placed her in the hands of doctors and nurses I had known for a few minutes, yet, I truly trusted them with my own beloved mother. This was not happenstance, this was the love created by God. The love that always trusts and is not boastful. When things went wrong at her unit and I forgave mistakes, I had realized that this was an Alzheimer's world now and I needed to be accepting and less judgmental. This was the love that kept no record of wrongs. When I trusted the advice of the courts, the medicine changes, and just held my breath praying I was making the right decision, that was the love that protects, always hopes. The day I turned my mommy over to the care of Hospice and said, "No more, let her go in peace," that was the day I thought I would die alongside her. But, this was pure love that does not dishonor others and is not self-seeking. The unconditional love between a mother and a daughter. I loved her enough to let her go. Love that always protects and rejoices in truths.

My mother taught me many things, her disease taught me everything I needed to know. Our journey through the mire of her disease made known to me the truest feelings of love from others to us - just as the sun imparts its warmth.

My thoughts and prayers are with any, and everyone who reads "Fading Image." Remember, there are many of us and we are not alone!

If I had faith that I could move mountains,
but didn't love others, I would be nothing.
1 Corinthians 13:2 NLT

Dallas Police Chief Billy Prince awarding Mom 25 year service pin. August 30, 1982. She would retire almost ten years later.

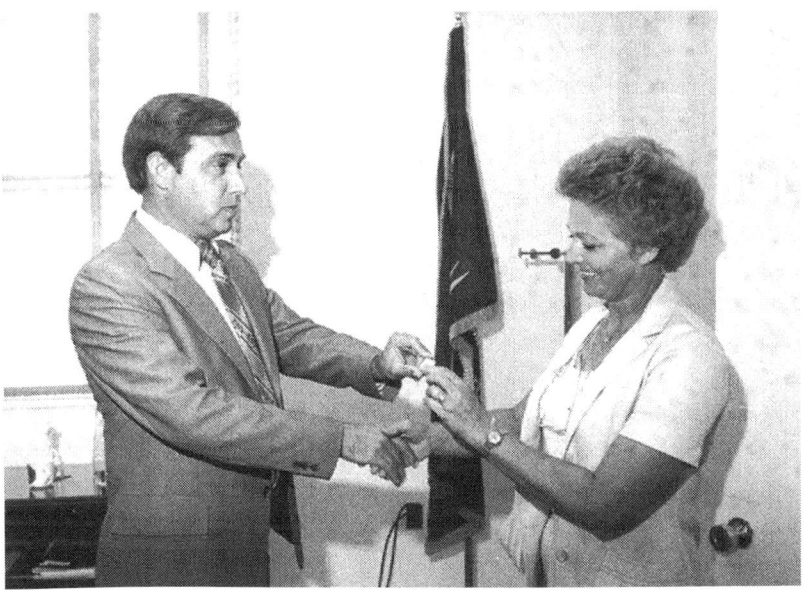

Rosemary "Rosie" Katzen

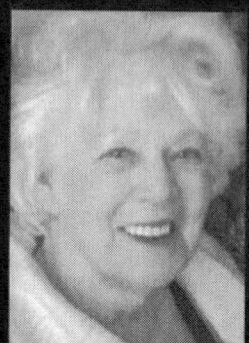

BORN: Monday December 3, 1934
DIED: Wednesday March 11, 2015

SERVICE

Sunday March 15, 2015
2:00 PM
Rest Haven Funeral Home - Rowlett Chapel
3701 Rowlett Rd.
Rowlett, TX 75088

Rosemary "Rosie" Katzen, age 80 of Rowlett, TX, passed away March 11, 2015. She was born December 3, 1934, in Malvern, AR, to Arch and Rosa (Reynolds) Dedman, the youngest of 9 children. Rosie grew up in Malvern where at the age of 14 she made her profession of Christian faith in Taylor's Chapel and was baptized in a creek. In 1957 she was the 5th female to join the Dallas Police Department and wore Badge #2071. Rosie retired in 1990 as Lieutenant. She was tough, but loving and was highly involved with the community. A member of First Rowlett United Methodist Church, she volunteered in mission work painting houses and gardening, and she was a talented seamstress. Rosie's hobbies were traveling, bunco and cards. She was dearly loved by family, neighbors and friends and will be greatly missed.

Mom receiving her 25 year pin with the DPD. made this quilt for me with my momma's scarves.

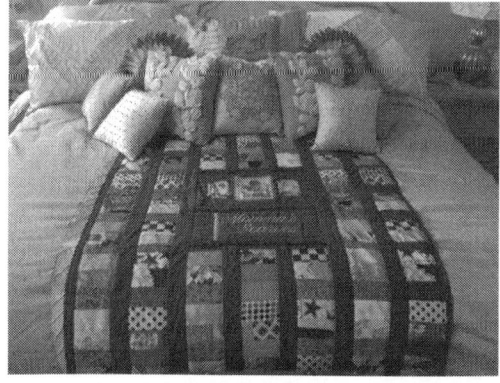

Fading Image

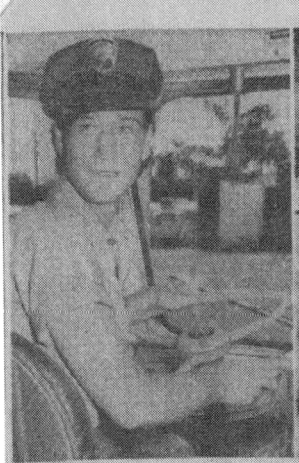 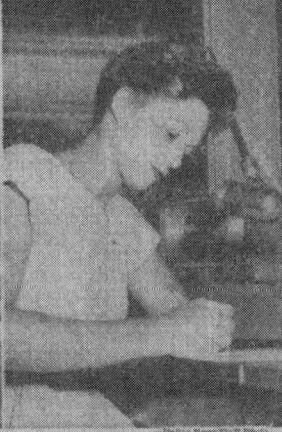

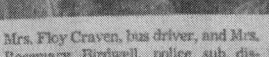

Mrs. Floy Craven, bus driver, and Mrs. Rosemary Birdwell, police sub dispatcher, are Dallas women holding down manly jobs in man's (?) world.

— Dallas News Staff Photo

IT'S A WOMAN'S WORLD, AT LEAST IN SOME JOBS

By DON KNOLES

Precisely on time at 8:12 a.m. one day this week, a White Rock Express bus roared bravely down... rolled boldly into the early-morning traffic rush on Garland Road.

A motorist, stopped for the light, did an appreciative double-take as the driver wheeled the big bus expertly on its way, for the driver was a woman.

While the feminine side has undisputedly taken its place on many such jobs, the gaping motorist was proof that this still comes as a surprise to a lot of males.

The driver, Mrs. Floy Craven, is among the ranks of Dallas women who not only bring home the bacon but also go out into a man's world to do it.

Mrs. Craven said her salary is not only better than most women's but also equivalent to her husband's. He is a driver of a moving van.

One of six women drivers for the Dallas Transit Company; she knows how to drive all buses in the barn—trolleys and diesel and gasoline buses.

She has no patience with the idea that she may be intruding into an exclusive male occupation. "I never think about it on those terms," she said. "Women should learn to take care of themselves, at the same time men ought to learn how to cook their own eggs at home."

Mrs. Craven, 32, who has been driving buses for nine months and...

has yet to have an accident that could have been prevented by herself, explained that she took the bus-driver job because she "hated being cooped indoors."

Cooped indoors, but also encroaching on the hereditle sacred working sanctuary of the male, is Mrs. Inge Bentgen, barber at De George's Barber Shop.

A barber for 11 years, she admitted that men had refused to get into her chair—although this has happened only twice. Once in Germany and once in Dallas.

Mrs. Bentgen, 27, a barber in Germany for seven years and in Dallas for four years, may receive some apprehension, but little trouble from her male customers.

"They rarely get fresh," she said. "They can't afford to. I've got the razor and scissors."

She finds it hard to give "Beatop" haircuts. "At first," she said, "I didn't have the heart to cut their hair so short. In Germany men like their hair long. But over here it's a lot hotter and the shorter haircut is more comfortable."

When a woman's voice first broke over the Dallas police radio, some of the older hands showed resentment, but Mrs. Rosemary Birdwell, 23, persisted and her voice is now a familiar sound over the hard-boiled frequency.

One of several women who sub as dispatchers along with male counterparts, the feels that woman's voices carry better than men's over the air.

She is the mother of a 6-year-old daughter.

Mrs. Birdwell agrees that the man's world has been cracked by the female and, characteristically, the male is sometimes bewildered. "But after all," says Mrs. Birdwell, "Aren't the women taking over?"

Illness Delays Steel Hearing

A court hearing concerning the strike last fall at the Lone Star Steel Company in Daingerfield was postponed Wednesday because of Dist. Judge W. L. Jack Thornton's illness.

The hearing is an injunction suit brought for 850 new employees who face the loss of their jobs when strikers are reinstated. Strikers were "fired" last Sept. 23 but the company accepted an arbitrator's decision last week to reinstate them.

The hearing is scheduled to resume Thursday.

Burrus Contracts

Contracts have been awarded to Burrus Mills, Inc., of Dallas to process commodity credit corporation-owned wheat into 2,436,600 pounds of flour, the Washington Bureau of The News reported Wednesday. The flour will be used for donation to domestic outlets such as school lunch programs, institutions and welfare agencies, the Agriculture Department reported.

The Dallas Morni

Local News . Editorial . Financi
DALLAS, TEXAS, THURSDAY,

Hearing Air
Precinct Tiff

By BILL GLINES

Dallas County Democrats proved again Wednesday night that there are two things they dearly like to do:

1. Vote.
2. Fight about it afterwards.

Charges of locking out voters at precinct conventions, fist fights and running off with voter lists were aired at a meeting of the party's credentials committee in Judge Owen Giles' courtroom in the Records Building.

After two hours of debate the credentials committee OK'd delegate groups picked at four precinct conventions Saturday—three conservative, one liberal.

The lockout took place at Precinct 241, the Edward K. Kerr School area. Several persons complained they were unable to get in because the school doors were locked. Finally, some of them did. But they were voted back out.

Carlos Holston Jr., elected precinct chairman, admitted the lockout was tough on everyone.

"One of my floor leaders was locked out. One official locked out was my wife; another a next door neighbor."

Laurence Melton, who heads the committee, chided Holston, and said the lockout was improper.

Manuel DeBusk, the executive committee's executive secretary, said that in the future, convention...

officials would be instructed to allow delegates arriving to take part in activities.

A liberal delegation was seated in Precinct 160, Cumberland School. Conservatives grumbled when they said they were not given proper recognition.

Bill Hicke, representing a liberal faction in Precinct 315, Neely Bryan School, said 6 or 15 persons participating did not register or have their taxes examined.

"When I tried to get the list a man grabbed it from the convention secretary, ran outdoors and jumped into his car," Hicke said.

Convention officials said there was no material difference in the outcome of the vote.

The big ruckus was in Precinct 135, Plymouth Park School, during...

A. B. Nixon, a liberal, charged that persons who participated in the Republican primary earlier in the day may have taken part in the Democratic primary.

He said that when he challenged a 55-36 vote to elect Robert Nelson as permanent chairman, he was denied recognition. Finally, he added, the way he counted was 36-22 vote.

After this "physical act" broke loose when a couple began fighting.

Injuries Suffered in Wreck Prove Fatal to Irving Man

Marvin Gelwin, 45-year-old Irving truck driver, died Wednesday in Parkland Hospital from injuries received in a 2-car head-on collision near Irving Monday.

Gelwin, who lived at 105 Elm Fork in Irving, became the tenth fatality on county highways in 1958.

His car and a car driven by Harold R. Church, 29, collided one mile east of Irving on Highway 183. Church was not injured.

Meanwhile, two Dallas motorcyclists were reported in critical condition at Baylor Hospital Wednesday night with head and back injuries suffered when their motorcycle apparently went out of control on U.S. Highway 80 near Hutchins.

Injured were Maurice Miller, 24, of 3314 Southern Oaks, and Mike Wilson, 16, of 3420 Southern Oaks.

Another motorcyclist, John Bridges, 45, of 308 Hillcrest, Richardson, remained in serious condition at Baylor Hospital suffering head injuries. The motorcyclist when his motorcycle struck gravel and went out of control at Arapaho and Greenville.

And a 25-year-old Dallas woman who was injured in an accident late Tuesday at Highway 183 and Belt Line Road, remained in critical condition.

Mrs. Lelia Cathey, of 1306 Drive, was a passenger in her husband's car when it collided with a truck.

227

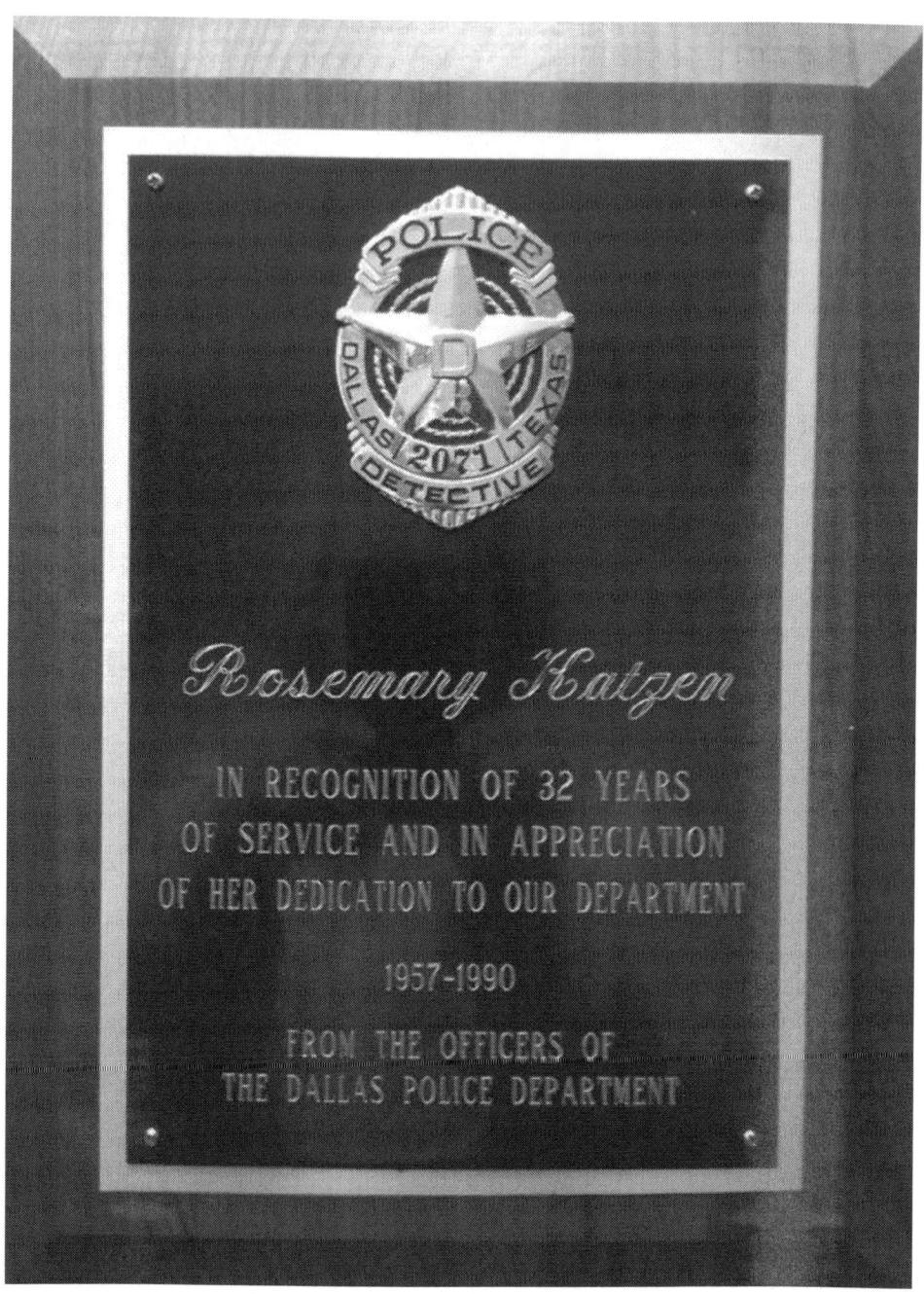

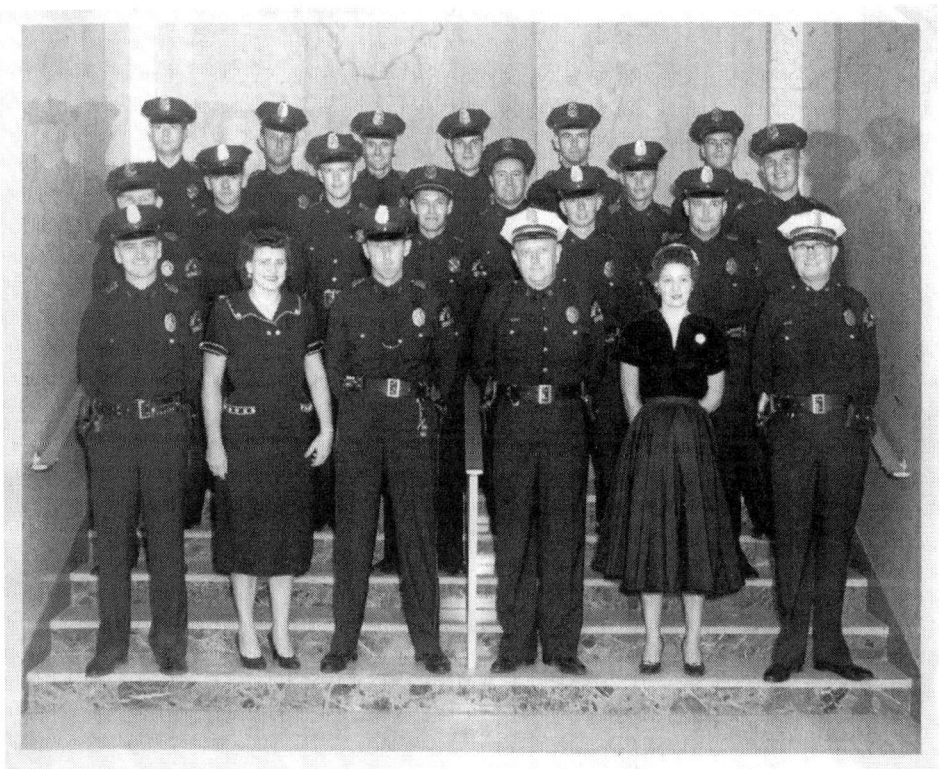

Mom in her police academy picture in 1957 (front row far right)

Rosemary Dedman Katzen Retirement 1990, Dallas Police Department

- 32 years of service, just 12 days short of 33 years
- 1957 started as a civilian as one of the first female dispatchers for DPD
- 1965 to 1973 she was a policewoman working the Juvenile division (now youth division)
- 1973 to 1974 she worked in the DA's office
- 1974 to 1975 she worked in Burglary and Theft division
- 1975 to 1982 she worked Special Investigations. During that time she recovered over two million dollars in missing property, and received the Certificate of **Merit.** This was all stolen property and did not include any drugs.
- 1982 to retirement:

    She worked in the Forgery Unit.

    She was one of the top investigators.

    She accumulated over 18 accommodations

    She achieved award for 25 years of safe driving

    She was considered an Outstanding Officer

About The Author

Mary believes there is a writer in each of us. She cannot remember a time when she was not writing. Words are like manna to her. Give her a Dictionary and a Thesaurus and she is in Heaven. She truly believes her writing talent is a gift from her Creator. Poems come so easily, most written within a fifteen minute period. She feels the words before they become a poem or an idea. Mary feels anything written from the heart is just feelings transposed onto thoughts on paper; like seeds planted and budding from the earth.

Her poem *It was never enough* written in 2002 became a song for the group FOR-GIVEN and on their CD, Forgiven by Request. She was asked to write something for one of the group members who was celebrating his 20th wedding anniversary. She wrote the poem on the way home from work at stop lights. She just felt how a man and a woman should love one another. As though it was never enough. When she called to share the poem with the Forgiven group leader, he implied he already had the music in his head for it. The poem became the song and it was never enough was created.

In 2010 Mary began the often dispirited journey along the road of Alzheimer's with her mother. Writing became her greatest outlet. A blog of feelings on FB, sometimes daily. She found there were others, in fact many, who shared her same feelings of help-lessness with a sick loved one. Sharing gave her solace over the years. In 2015 after her mother passed away she was prodded by many to share her experience and love by writing a book. At first she would just write a story of her time with her mother and then she decided if people wanted to really feel what care giving was like, the good and the bad, she would publish the blog and a few chapters to go with it.

Thus the book, *Fading Image* was created. A little about the disease of Alzheimer's, a lot more about love and faith.

Mary lives in Texas and is blessed to be surrounded by friends and family as she pro-gresses through her grieving process. She continues to write and hopes to publish a children's book next....*Teacups and Radishes*, a comical poem about a tea party with teacups and radishes. Mary can be found at maryraybirdwell.com
Mary Ray Birdwell

References

National Institute of Neurological Disorders and Stroke.
Ninds.nih.gov (2016, February 2) Retrieved February 3rd, 2016 from
http://www.ninds.nih.gov/disorders/alzheimersdisease/alzheimersdisease.htm

Alzheimer's disease
mayoclinic.org (2015, December 22nd)
Retrieved January 1st, 2016 from http://www.mayoclinic.org/diseases-conditions/alz-heimers-disease/home/ovc-20167098

Alzheimer's disease: Symptoms, Stages, Diagnosis and Coping Tips.
www.helpguide (2016, February) Retrieved February 2016 from http://www.help-guide.org/articles/alzheimers-dementia/alzheimers-disease.htm

Diagnosis of Alzheimer's Disease and Dementia www.Alz.org (2016) Retrieved January 2nd, 2016 from http://www.alz.org/alzheimers_disease_diagnosis.asp

Made in the USA
Charleston, SC
18 May 2016